THROMBOSIS, ATHEROSCLEROSIS AND ATHEROTHROMBOSIS - NEW INSIGHTS AND EXPERIMENTAL PROTOCOLS

Edited by **Mojca Božič-Mijovski**

Thrombosis, Atherosclerosis and Atherothrombosis - New Insights and Experimental Protocols
http://dx.doi.org/10.5772/59831
Edited by Mojca Božič-Mijovski

Contributors

Jasmina Dragan Dimitrova-Shumkovska, Snezna Sodin-Semrl, Polona Žigon, Mojca Božič-Mijovski, Mojca Frank Bertoncelj, Saša Čučnik, Matija Tomšič, Aleš Ambrožič, Borut Božič, Tanja Kveder, Alojzija Hočevar, Atsushi Yamashita, Christos Yapijakis, Vinko Boc, Vladka Salapura, Aleš Blinc, Mojca Stegnar, Rita Rezzani, Francesca Bonomini, Gaia Favero

Published by InTech

Janeza Trdine 9, 51000 Rijeka, Croatia

Publishing Process Manager Iva Lipovic

Technical Editor InTech DTP team

Cover InTech Design team

First published December, 2015

Printed in Croatia

Additional hard copies can be obtained from orders@intechopen.com

Thrombosis, Atherosclerosis and Atherothrombosis - New Insights and Experimental Protocols, Edited by Mojca Božič-Mijovski

p. cm.

ISBN 978-953-51-2226-5

For EU product safety concerns:
IN TECH d.o.o., Prolaz Marije Krucifikse Kozulić 3, 51000 Rijeka, Croatia,
info@intechopen.com or visit our website at intechopen.com.

Meet the editor

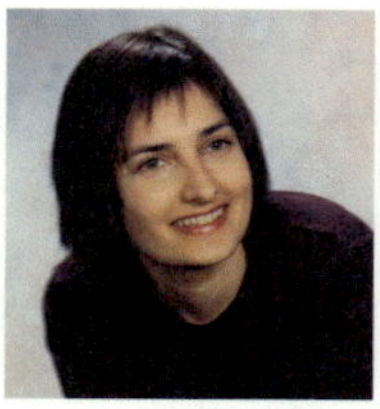

Dr. Mojca Božič-Mijovski is the Head of Laboratory for Haemostasis and Thrombosis at the University Medical Centre, Ljubljana, and is Assistant Professor in Haemostasis at the University of Ljubljana, Faculty of Pharmacy. She received her PhD in Biochemistry and Molecular Biology at the Medical Faculty (University of Ljubljana) and specialist degree in Medical Biochemistry at the Slovenian Ministry of Health. She is a member of the Scientific Board of the European and Mediterranean League against Thrombotic Diseases, member of the International Society of Thrombosis and Haemostasis and President of the Commission for Continuous Education at the Slovene Chamber of Laboratory Medicine. Her research in the field of thrombosis and haemostasis resulted in almost 30 articles published in peer-reviewed journals.

Contents

Preface

Thrombosis is a result of thrombus formation on a disrupted plaque that leads to acute myocardial infarction or stroke. However, atherosclerotic plaque disruption does not always result in acute thrombotic events. This book starts with a review on thrombus growth pathophysiology. Atherosclerosis, however, progresses silently over several decades. Current evidence supports a central role of inflammatory signalling pathways in the initiation, progression and thrombotic complications of atherosclerosis. In the second chapter of this book, the role of the major transcription factor – nuclear factor kappa B (NF-kB) – is elucidated, which is involved in the transcription of many genes with an established role in atherosclerosis and regulation of many functions of the vessel wall.

Translocator protein (TSPO), located in the outer mitochondrial membrane, is involved in cholesterol metabolism, inflammation, oxidative stress response and other (non-atherosclerotic) processes. The third chapter presents an in-depth study on the associations between TSPO and elevated levels of cholesterol and platelet count, both known risk factors of thrombosis. TSPO is presented as a novel therapeutic target and diagnostic tool for research on cardiovascular diseases and their complications.

Besides inflammation, coagulation plays a pivotal role in the pathogenesis of vascular disease, and there is an extensive cross-talk between both systems. Inflammation leads to coagulation activation, and coagulation considerably affects inflammatory activity. In the fourth chapter, the current and emerging biomarkers of hypercoagulability and inflammation are discussed, followed by a presentation of the role of these markers as predictors of restenosis after percutaneous transluminal angioplasty. The last two chapters deal with hypercoagulability caused by thrombophilic factors – antiphospholipid bodies and common gene polymorphisms associated with thrombophilia.

This book offers a broad, contemporary review of atherosclerotic processes that lead to thrombosis. In addition, it includes experimental protocols, by which these processes are studied, providing the reader with the information necessary to understand the complexity of the disease process and the current experimental methodology in finding new answers that would help in the diagnosis, prevention and treatment of atherosclerotic disease.

Mojca Božič-Mijovski
Laboratory for Haemostasis and Atherothrombosis
Department of Vascular Diseases
University Medical Centre Ljubljana
Ljubljana, Slovenia

Chapter 1

Pathophysiology of Atherothrombosis — Thrombus Growth, Vascular Thrombogenicity, and Plaque Metabolism

Atsushi Yamashita and Yujiro Asada

Additional information is available at the end of the chapter

http://dx.doi.org/10.5772/61769

Abstract

Atherosclerotic plaque disruption does not always result in acute symptomatic events. Therefore, the formation of a large thrombus is a critical step in the development of atherothrombosis. However, little is known about the mechanisms involved in thrombus growth processes after plaque disruption. Studies in vivo have demonstrated that the tissue factor (TF) derived from the vascular wall contributes to the formation of thrombin-dependent platelet–fibrin thrombus on atherosclerotic arteries but not on normal arteries, and that altered blood flow in disrupted atherosclerotic arteries promotes platelet recruitment mediated by von Willebrand factor (VWF) on the thrombus surface and augmented blood coagulation resulting in thrombus growth. The thrombogenic potential of plaques is a fundamental factor in atherothrombosis. We recently found that the arterial glucose uptake reflects vascular thrombogenicity, which might be partly explained by metabolic adaptation and enhanced procoagulant activity in a hypoxic microenvironment. Hypoxic responses might link atherometabolism to vascular thrombogenicity.

Keywords: Atherometabolism, hypoxia, plaque erosion, thrombus growth, plaque thrombogenicity

1. Introduction

Thrombus formation on a ruptured or an eroded atherosclerotic plaque is a critical event that leads to atherothrombosis. However, autopsy studies have identified asymptomatic coronary thrombi on disrupted plaques and pathological differences in plaques with symptomatic and asymptomatic thrombi [1, 2]. Therefore, plaque disruption is not a final step, whereas thrombus growth processes are critical for the development of atherothrombosis. Despite intensive investigation into the mechanisms of atherogenesis and plaque instability [3], little is known about the mechanisms involved in thrombus growth after plaque disruption. Vascular thrombogenicity and changes in blood flow and blood factors are generally thought to regulate thrombus formation. Therefore, disparities in these regulators affect the thrombus growth, and atherosclerotic plaque thrombogenicity is an essential factor for atherothrombosis. Plaque vulnerability, the upregulation of prothrombotic factors, and the downregulation of antithrombotic factors in atherosclerotic plaques have been demonstrated [3–5], and inflammatory stimuli play important roles in plaque thrombogenicity [6]. However, the determinants of vascular wall thrombogenicity are not fully understood.

Arterial inflammation has been evaluated using positron emission tomography (PET) imaging with [^{18}F]-fluorodeoxyglucose (^{18}F-FDG). The close correlation between ^{18}F-FDG uptake and plaque macrophage contents in animal models of atherosclerosis [7] suggests that the degree of ^{18}F-FDG reflects the underlying levels of vascular inflammation. Clinical studies have identified a relationship between ^{18}F-FDG uptake and numbers of cardiovascular risk factors, as well as risk for future events [8, 9]. The uptake of ^{18}F-FDG is significantly higher in aortic segments with thrombus than without thrombus in a rabbit model of advanced atherosclerosis [10]. These lines of evidence imply an association between glucose uptake and vascular thrombogenicity, although the underlying mechanism is unknown.

This article focuses on the pathophysiology of thrombus growth on disrupted plaques and discusses a conceivable relationship between atherometabolism and vascular thrombogenicity.

2. Pathology of atherothrombosis

Arterial thrombi are mainly composed of aggregated platelets as a likely result of rapid blood flow, and the development of platelet-rich thrombi is regarded as a cause of atherothrombosis. Fresh coronary thrombi in patients with acute myocardial infarction (AMI) and unstable angina have become assessable due to technological advances, distal protection, and thrombus aspiration devices. Evidence gathered from such studies indicates that such fresh atherothrombi consist of aggregated platelets, fibrin, erythrocytes, and white blood cells comprising mostly neutrophils, and that they are constitutively immunopositive for the platelet integrin αIIbβ3, fibrin, the membrane protein expressed on erythrocytes glycophorin A, and the von Willebrand factor (VWF; blood adhesion molecule). VWF and tissue factor (TF; initiator of the coagulation cascade) are closely associated with integrin αIIbβ3 and fibrin, respectively [11, 12] (Figure 1). These findings suggest that the enhanced platelet aggregation and fibrin formation result in thrombus growth and obstructive thrombus formation on disrupted atherosclerotic plaques, and that VWF and/or TF contribute to the pathological process.

Pathological findings suggest that plaque disruption and sudden coronary occlusion are often preceded by a variable period of thrombus formation. Aspirated thrombi from one-third to half of patients with AMI show cell lytic changes and/or organizing reactions, namely endothelialization with or without smooth muscle cell (SMC) ingrowth [13, 14] (Figure 2).

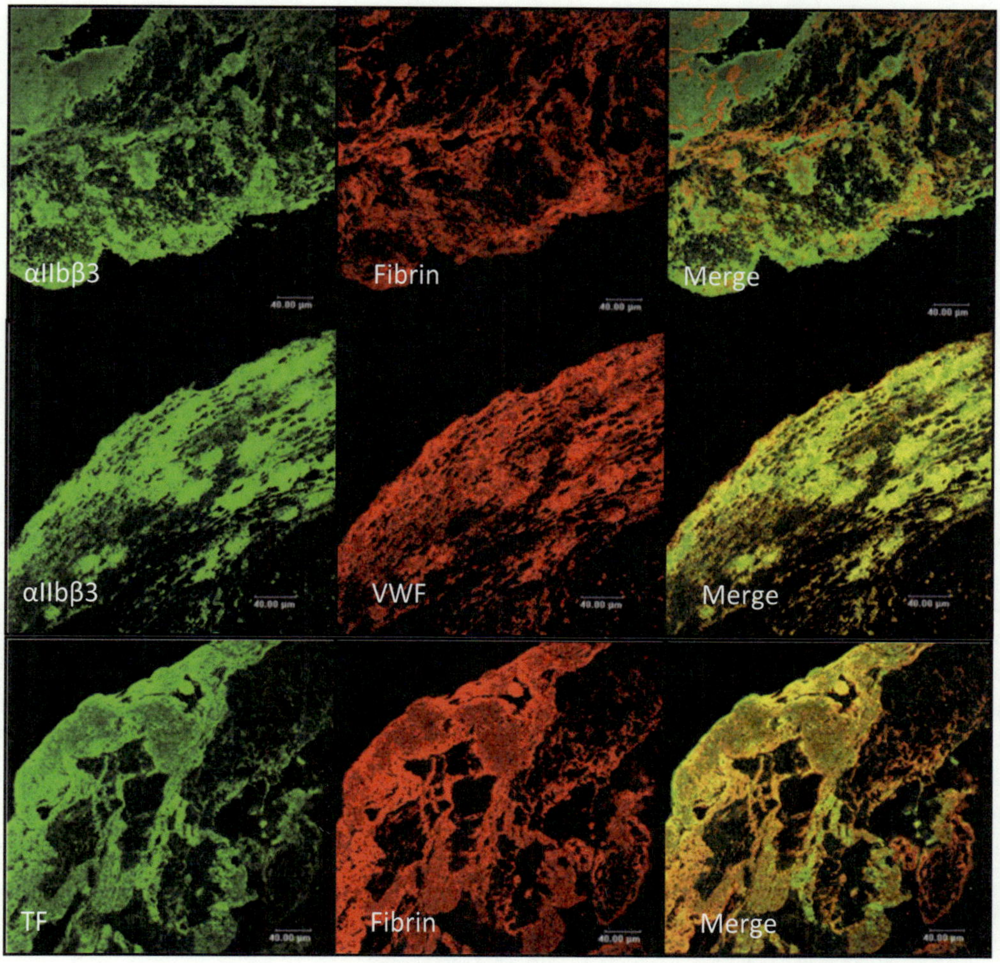

Figure 1. Immunofluorescence micrographs of fresh coronary thrombi in patients with acute myocardial infarction. Left, staining with fluorescein isothiocyanate-labeled integrin αIIbβ3, VWF, and TF (green). Center, staining with Cy3 labeled with fibrin and VWF (red). Right, merged immunofluorescence images. Areas of colocalized factors are stained yellow. Atherothrombus comprises platelets and fibrin. VWF and TF are closely associated with αIIbβ3 and fibrin, respectively. TF, tissue factor; VWF von Willebrand factor (from Ref. 11 with permission).

These findings indicate that the thrombi are aged more than several days after formation. In addition, organizing thrombus is associated with the in-hospital and long-term mortality of patients with AMI [14, 15].

Plaques become disrupted via rupture and erosion. Plaques rupture when a thin fibrous cap ruptures, which allows blood to come in contact with a thrombogenic necrotized core, resulting in thrombus formation. A ruptured plaque is characterized by disrupted thin fibrous caps, usually < 65 μm thick, abundant macrophages and lymphocytes, and a few SMCs [16]. Thus, a thinning fibrous cap is thought to represent a state that is vulnerable to rupture, which is referred to as thin-cap fibroatheroma [17]. However, this is not taken into account in the current

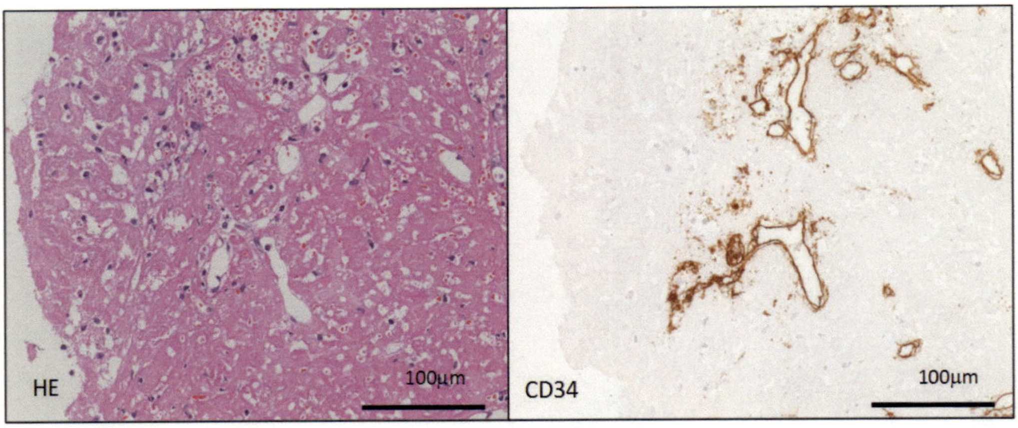

Figure 2. Light and immunohistochemical images of acute coronary thrombi in patients with acute myocardial infarction. Thrombus comprises degraded erythrocytes and leukocytes, mononuclear cell infiltrate, and small luminal structures lined with flat or spindle cells. CD34 immunostaining highlights endothelialization and microvessel formation in the thrombus, indicating organized reaction, even acute onset of AMI. HE, hematoxylin eosin stain.

American Heart Association classification of atherosclerosis. Plaques undergoing erosion are characterized by a denuded surface and thrombus formation, and lack a disrupted fibrous cap. Patients with plaque erosion are younger and are not predominantly males compared with those who have ruptured plaques. Angiography has shown that the luminal surface of eroded plaques is less narrowed and irregular. The morphological features include abundant SMCs and proteoglycan matrix, especially versican and hyaluronan, and disrupted surface endothelium. An eroded plaque contains relatively few macrophages and T cells compared with a ruptured plaque [16]. In contrast, macrophages comprise the dominant cell type at sites of both plaque rupture and erosion, and both inflammatory cells and SMCs express human leukocyte antigen (HLA-DR) antigens [18]. These findings suggest that eroded plaques are heterogeneous and that both inflammatory and noninflammatory processes contribute to the development of plaque erosion. The proportions of fibrin and platelets differ in coronary thrombi on ruptured and eroded plaques. Thrombi on ruptured and eroded plaques are rich in fibrin and platelets, respectively. The tissue factor is abundant in a ruptured plaque compared with an eroded plaque [19]. These characteristics of ruptured and eroded plaques (abundant TF, phospholipids, and less matrix protein in ruptured sites; abundant matrix protein and less TF in eroded sites) might explain the difference in the composition of thrombi in ruptured and eroded plaques.

3. Pathology of asymptomatic plaque disruption

Clinical angioscopy studies have revealed that asymptomatic multiple plaque rupture is a frequent complication among patients with coronary atherothrombosis [20]. Various stages of healed plaque disruption are also occasionally found during autopsies of individuals with and without known coronary atherothrombosis [2, 21]. Hearts at autopsy from patients who died

http://dx.doi.org/10.5772/61769

of AMI have been compared with hearts form those who succumbed to noncardiac death to determine the incidence and morphological characteristics of thrombi and plaque disruption in patients with noncardiac death [1]. This study found coronary thrombi in 16% of noncardiac deaths; most of them had developed an eroded plaque and were too small to affect the coronary lumen (Figure 3). Smaller lipid areas, thicker fibrous caps, and more modest luminal narrowing were features of disrupted plaques associated with noncardiac death compared with AMI. Davies et al. [21] and Arbustini et al. [22] found coronary thrombus in 4% and 7% of noncardiac deaths, respectively, at autopsy. The coronary thrombi from noncardiac deaths were associated with eroded plaques [22]. These results suggest that plaque disruption does not always result in complete thrombotic occlusion with subsequent acute symptomatic events, and that thrombus growth is a critical step in the onset of clinical events. However, the determinants of coronary thrombus size after plaque disruption remain unknown.

The histological assessment of 157 carotid endarterectomy samples from asymptomatic patients and those with symptomatic major stroke revealed less frequent erosion in both symptomatic (3.1%) and asymptomatic plaques (6.7%) [23]. Less disrupted plaques, fewer inflammatory cells, a smaller necrotic core, and more calcification were identified in thrombotic plaques from the asymptomatic patients [23]. Because information about asymptomatic plaque disruption is limited, the features of coronary and carotid plaques are not identical.

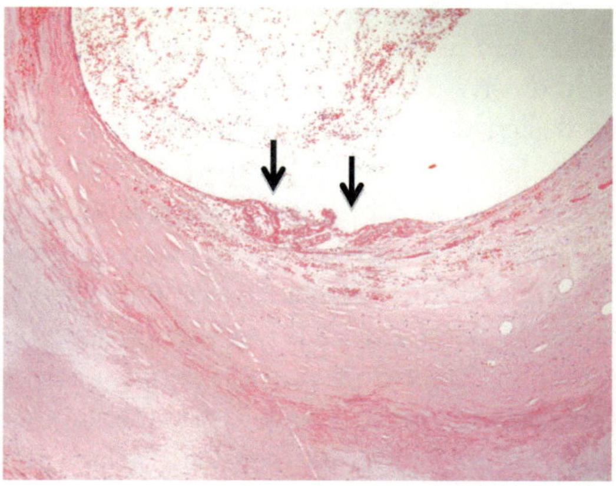

Figure 3. Coronary plaque erosion in patients with noncardiac death. Superficial erosive injury and mural thrombus (arrows) are evident on atherosclerotic lesions. A thrombus is too small to obstruct the coronary lumen and induce symptomatic events. HE, hematoxylin eosin stain (from Ref. 1, with permission).

4. Pathophysiology of atherothrombosis

Atherothrombosis is initiated by plaque rupture or erosion. Accumulating evidence supports the notion that inflammation and matrix degradation contribute to plaque destabilization and that subsequent rupture of the fibrous cap triggers thrombus formation. Because the pathophysiology underlying plaque rupture is established [3], the pathophysiology of plaque erosion and thrombus growth is the focus of this section.

4.1. Possible mechanism of plaque erosion

Eroded plaque is characterized by a superficial plaque injury, but the mechanisms of such erosions are poorly understood. Approximately 80% thrombi associated with plaque erosion is nonocclusive regardless of sudden coronary death [16]. Experimental aortic stenosis can induce acute endothelial changes or damage to the normal aorta [24]. Therefore, hemodynamic forces, particularly those generated by disturbed blood flow induced by stenosis or vasoconstriction, could be a crucial factor in generating surface vascular damage and thrombosis. We investigated pathological changes after acute luminal narrowing in SMC-rich plaques in rabbits to understand the relationship between disturbed blood flow and plaque erosion. Balloon-induced injury of rabbit femoral arteries resulted in the formation of SMC-rich plaques comprising stellate- or spindle-shaped SMCs and extracellular matrix [25]. Acute vascular narrowing disrupted the blood flow in these arteries that consequently induced superficial erosive injury of the SMC-rich plaque. Figure 4 shows microscopic images of a longitudinal section of neointima at the post-stenotic region 15 min after vascular narrowing. The endothelial cells and SMCs at this region are broadly detached and associated with platelet adhesion to the subendothelium and a change in the shape of the SMCs. Endothelial cells and superficial SMCs became apoptotic within 15 min [26]. Subsequent vascular narrowing induced mural thrombi comprising platelets and fibrin, as in human plaque erosion. Thus, disrupted blood flow can induce superficial erosive damage to SMC-rich plaques and subsequent thrombus formation. We therefore designed a computational fluid simulation using the Reynolds-averaged Navier–Stokes model and calculated wall shear stress (WSS), turbulence kinetic energy (TKE), blood pressure, and blood pressure gradients (BPG) in a rabbit model to clarify the contribution of hemodynamic factors to the onset of plaque erosion in the SMC-rich plaque. The magnitude of WSS, TKE, and BPG correlated with the extent of histologically defined erosive damage. The values for WSS and TKE were significantly larger at eroded, than at noneroded sites [27]. Although direct clinical evidence has not supported the notion that coronary artery vasospasm plays a role in plaque erosion, ergonovine and norepinephrine-stimulated vasospasm of the atherosclerotic coronary artery has induced superficially damaged plaques and acute ischemic injury to the myocardium of a strain of Watanabe heritable hyperlipidemic rabbits that are prone to myocardial infarction [28]. Platelet and blood coagulation are activated in the coronary circulation after vasospastic angina [29, 30]. Although additional evidence is needed, hemodynamic factors might play an important role in the development of plaque erosion.

4.2. Thrombus growth and stability on disrupted plaques

Thrombus growth is considered critical to the onset of clinical events. Vascular wall thrombogenicity, local blood flow, and blood contents regulate thrombus formation, and thus thrombus growth seems to vary depending on the status of these three regulators. Nevertheless, a thrombogenic atherosclerotic lesion is essential for atherothrombosis.

http://dx.doi.org/10.5772/61769

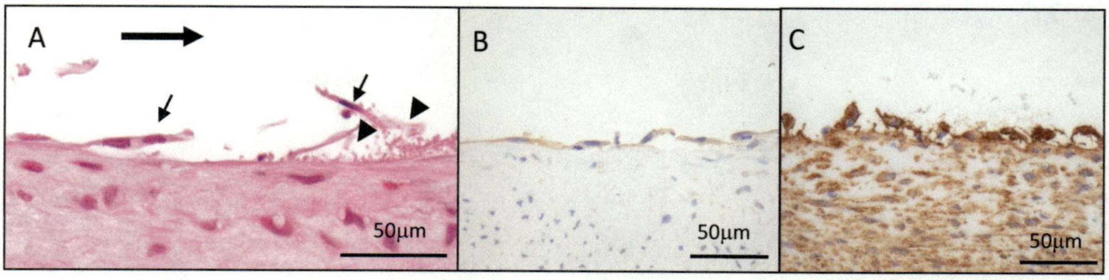

Figure 4. Representative images of the superficial erosive injury of SMC-rich plaques and thrombus formation. Smooth muscle cell-rich plaque 15 min after vascular narrowing shows endothelial detachment (small arrows) accompanied by platelet adhesion (arrow heads) at 1 mm from a region of vascular narrowing (A, hematoxylin eosin stain). Larger arrow indicates flow direction. Immunohistochemistry for VWF (marker of endothelium; B) and smooth muscle actin (marker of SMC; C) confirms detached endothelial cells and SMCs at the post-stenotic region (from Ref. 26).

The TF is overexpressed and its procoagulant activity is increased in human atherosclerotic plaques, and macrophages and SMC both express TF in the intima. The TF is more prominent in fatty streaks and atheromatous plaques than in a human aorta with diffuse intimal thickening [4]. Vascular wall TF appears to contribute to the size of thrombi on atherosclerotic lesions. On the other hand, studies in vitro have shown that not only monocytes but also neutrophils, eosinophils, and even platelets can synthesize TF. Although TF expression by blood cells remains controversial, monocytes are the only blood cells that are known to synthesize and express TF [31]. Plasma TF levels are elevated in patients with unstable angina and AMI and correlate with adverse outcomes [32]. Hematopoietic cell-derived, TF-positive microparticles contribute to laser injury-induced thrombosis in the microvasculature of the mouse cremaster muscle [33]. In contrast, vascular smooth muscle-derived TF contributes to thrombosis-induced $FeCl_3$ in the mouse carotid artery [34]. Therefore, whether vascular wall and/or blood-derived TF support thrombus propagation is controversial. We compared the contribution of plaques and/or blood TF with thrombus formation in the rabbit femoral artery with or without atherosclerotic lesions induced by a diet containing 0.5% cholesterol and balloon injury. We found TF expression and increased procoagulant activity in the atherosclerotic arteries compared with the normal femoral arteries. Balloon injury of the atherosclerotic plaque induced thrombin-dependent, large thrombi composed of platelet–fibrin. In contrast, balloon injury of normal femoral arteries induced thrombin-independent small platelet thrombi (Figure 5). Moreover, the whole-blood coagulation in rabbits was not affected by inhibiting the blood TF even under hyperlipidemic conditions [35]. Therefore, at least, atherosclerotic plaque-derived TF contributes to the activation of the intravascular coagulation cascade and to thrombus size on atherosclerotic lesions.

The tissue factor pathway inhibitor and argatroban, a thrombin inhibitor, reduce both platelet and fibrin content in atherosclerotic arteries but not in normal femoral arteries [35]. Oral-activated factor X (FXa) inhibitors significantly reduce the atherothrombus growth induced by balloon injury and vascular ligation in rabbits, and plasma FXa activity correlates with the antithrombotic effects of the oral FXa inhibitors [36]. These findings indicate that excess

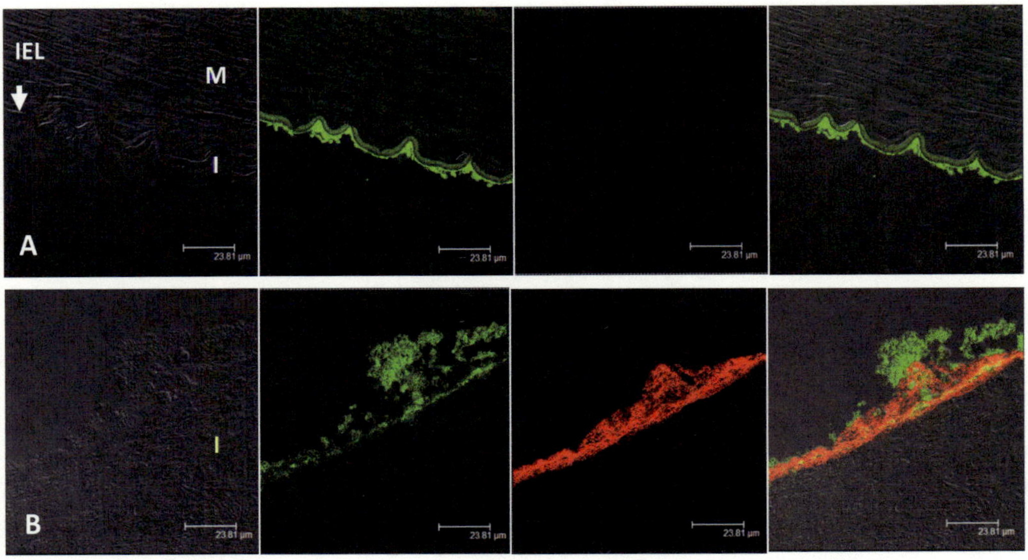

Figure 5. Immunofluorescence images of thrombus on rabbit femoral artery. Immunofluorescence microphotographs of thrombi 15 min after balloon injury of a normal femoral artery and of an atherosclerotic plaque under 0.5% cholesterol diet. Rows show differential interference contrast images, images stained with fluorescein isothiocyanate-labeled integrin αIIbβ3 (green), Cy3-labeled fibrin (red), and merged immunofluorescence images. Areas with colocalized factors are stained yellow. Thrombi on normal intima comprise small aggregated platelets (A), whereas large thrombi on atherosclerotic plaques comprise platelets and fibrin (B). I, intima; IEL, internal elastic lamina, M, media (from Ref. 35, with permission).

thrombin generation via FXa contributes to further platelet accumulation and fibrin formation on disrupted plaques. The FXa is generated by factor VII (FVII) or activated factor IX. The feedback activation of factors VIII and XI (FXI) by thrombin amplifies further thrombin generation through FXI-, FIX-, and FX activation (Figure 6). The intrinsic coagulation pathway is initiated when the coagulation factor XII (FXII) comes in contact with collagen, nucleic acids and polyphosphate, high-molecular mass kininogen, and plasma kallikrein. Factor XI is activated by activated FXII, thrombin, and activated XI (FXIa) in vitro [37]; it is present in platelet–fibrin thrombus induced by balloon injury of atherosclerotic lesions in rabbits, and anti-FXI antibody reduces thrombus formation without prolonging bleeding [38]. Factors XI and FXII do not affect the initial phase of thrombus formation but prevent thrombus shedding and contribute to thrombus stability on carotid ruptured plaques in ApoE-deficient mice [39, 40]. In contrast, the inhibition of activated FVII participates in the initial stage of thrombus formation on ruptured plaques [40]. These findings suggest that after plaque disruption, FXII- and FXI-mediated amplification of thrombin generation plays an important role in thrombus stability on disrupted plaques. However, a clinical study discovered an inverse relationship between levels of FXII and risk of myocardial infarction [41]. A deficiency of FXI did not prevent the development of acute coronary events [42] but reduced the incidence of deep vein thrombosis and ischemic strokes [43, 44]. The role of the intrinsic coagulation pathway in atherothrombosis requires further investigation.

http://dx.doi.org/10.5772/61769

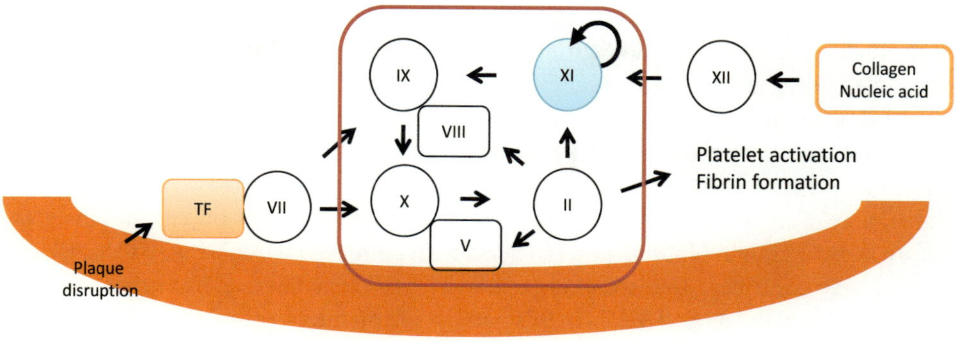

Figure 6. Exposure of prothrombotic factors and amplification of coagulation cascade on disrupted plaques. Exposure of the tissue factor, (TF) after plaque disruption, initiates blood coagulation. The activated factor X is generated by activated factors VII or IX. Feedback activation of factors VIII and XI by thrombin amplifies further thrombin generation through sequential activation of factors XI, IX, and X. Factor XI is also activated by intrinsic coagulation factor XII and activated factor XI. The excess thrombin generation via the feedback activation and intrinsic pathway contributes to further platelet accumulation and fibrin formation on disrupted plaques. Red square indicates platelet surface.

Platelets comprise a major cellular component in coronary thrombus and play an important role in not only the initial but also the growth phase of thrombus formation. Platelet recruitment to the thrombus surface and the stabilization of platelet activation are important to maintain platelet accumulation and thrombus growth. Adhesion molecules and their receptors on platelets are essential for thrombus formation, because they support platelet tethering and firm adhesion, as well as platelet aggregation and recruitment to the thrombus surface. The large, multimeric, plasma protein VWF undergoes a conformational change when bound to extracellular matrix and platelet surface, and the conformational change permits its binding to GPIbα. Studies in vitro and in vivo have shown that platelet recruitment to the thrombus surface is primarily mediated by VWF and GPIbα on flowing platelets [45, 46]. We found a large amount of VWF localized to coronary thrombi in patients with AMI [11], and that a monoclonal antibody against the VWF A1 domain that interacts with platelet GPIbα, significantly suppresses the formation of platelet–fibrin thrombi and completely inhibits the occlusive thrombus formation in rabbit atherosclerotic lesions [25, 47]. These findings indicate that VWF plays a crucial role in thrombus growth via platelet recruitment. Real-time analysis of platelet calcium flux during thrombus formation in vitro has shown that the stable adhesion between aggregated platelets and the growth of platelet thrombus depends on sustained integrin αIIbβ3 activation and cyclic calcium flux through secreted adenosine diphosphate and its $P2Y_1$ and $P2Y_{12}$ receptors [48, 49]. We administer anti-$P2Y_{12}$ antagonists to prevent secondary cardiovascular events because these drugs destabilize thrombus and limit thrombus formation.

4.3. Effects of altered blood flow on thrombus growth

Blood flow is a key modulator of thrombus growth, and coronary blood flow is altered in patients with ischemic heart diseases. Marzilli et al. [50] found that the coronary blood flow is reduced by about 80% during ischemia in patients with unstable angina and an autopsy study frequently found intramyocardial microemboli in patients who succumbed to sudden coronary death [51]. Distal microvascular embolism and/or vasoconstriction could affect blood flow as well as thrombus formation and growth at culprit lesions. We examined the effects of the blood flow reduction on thrombus formation in an animal model and found that > 75% reduction in blood flow promoted the growth of thrombus consisting of a mixture of platelets and fibrin on atherosclerotic lesions that subsequently became occlusive, and it also induced the formation of very small thrombi composed only of platelets on normal arteries [47]. Therefore, a reduction in blood flow associated with increased vascular wall thrombogenicity is considered to contribute to thrombus growth. We also identified an important role of the 5-HT_{2A} receptor on platelets and SMCs in this process via platelet aggregation and thrombogenic vasoconstriction [52, 53].

In addition to distal vascular resistance, blood flow disturbed by acute vascular narrowing promotes thrombus growth at post-stenotic regions. As described above, vascular narrowing of the rabbit femoral artery induced superficial erosive injury to SMC-rich plaque. The progression of neointimal damage caused by disturbed blood flow was associated with thrombus growth. These findings suggest that the degree of plaque disruption affects thrombus size after the plaque erosion [26].

The rheological effect on thrombus growth might be partly explained by a shear gradient-dependent mechanism of platelet aggregation. Nesbitt et al. [54] used imaging to reveal a shear gradient-dependent, platelet-aggregation process that is preceded by the soluble agonist-dependent aggregation in stenotic microvessels in vitro and in vivo. Shear microgradients at post-stenotic regions or downstream of thrombi induce stable platelet aggregates, the sizes of which are directly influenced by shear microgradients. This process requires ligand binding to integrin αIIbβ3 and transient Ca^{2+} flux, but does not require a change in global platelet shape or soluble agonists. These findings suggest that a biomechanical mechanism is principally involved in the early phase of platelet adhesion and aggregation. Vessel and/or thrombus geometry itself might promote thrombus formation.

Platelet and/or fibrin aggregates must exceed the physical forces exerted by blood flow within the narrowing lumen for thrombus to become occlusive and VWF is a candidate in the final process. The thrombogenic activity of VWF is strictly dependent upon its multimeric structure. A critical shear stress of 35 ± 3.5 dyn/cm^2 induces VWF to change from a globular state to an extended chain conformation [55]. Such excessive shear stress can induce platelet aggregation in the absence of exogenous agonists [56], and the interaction between VWF and platelets under high shear rates might be a key determinant of the final process of thrombotic occlusion. In fact, inhibiting the plasma VWF completely prevents occlusive thrombus formation induced by neointimal injury and disrupted blood flow in rabbits [47].

5. Atherometabolism and vascular wall thrombogenicity

Atherosclerotic plaque thrombogenicity is an essential factor for the development of atherothrombosis. However, the determinants of vascular wall thrombogenicity are not yet fully understood. Understanding the factors that reflect vascular wall thrombogenicity will allow the detection of high-risk plaques and the development of novel therapies for atherosclerosis that target vascular thrombogenicity.

Metabolism in higher animals including humans is finely regulated by metabolic organs, a neuroendocrine system, and cellular regulatory mechanisms. Recent studies have found that distinct metabolic states maintain the functions of cancerous and inflammatory cells within specific microenvironments [57, 58]. Because enhanced glucose metabolism has been visualized by ^{18}F-FDG-PET in some atherosclerotic lesions, we speculate that the metabolically active plaque is highly thrombogenic. Therefore, this section focuses on atherometabolism and vascular wall thrombogenicity.

5.1. Glucose uptake reflects vascular wall thrombogenicity

Although recent advances in clinical imaging have revealed detailed anatomical information about atherosclerotic lesions, functional information remains limited. The uptake of ^{18}F-FDG in atherosclerosis closely correlates with macrophage contents in rabbits [7]. Clinical studies have also found a relationship between ^{18}F-FDG uptake and future cardiovascular events [9, 59]. Thus, the evidence implies an association between ^{18}F-FDG uptake and arterial thrombus formation. We therefore visualized rabbit atherosclerotic and contralateral nonatherosclerotic femoral arteries using ^{18}F-FDG-PET, and induced arterial thrombus by balloon injury. The images revealed more radioactivity along the atherosclerotic than along the contralateral nonatherosclerotic artery. Areas of arterial thrombus correlated with the amount of arterial radioactivity determined from the PET images and autoradiography. The amount of arterial radioactivity positively correlated with macrophage contents, TF expression, and the nuclear localization of NF-κB, a transcriptional factor of TF. Inhibiting NF-κB reduced TF expression in rabbit atherosclerotic plaques cultured in vitro [60]. In addition, more ^{18}F-FDG is taken up by advanced atherosclerotic segments with thrombus induced by Russell's viper venom and histamine compared with segments without thrombus in the rabbit aorta [10]. An imaging study using apoE-deficient mice showed colocalization of deoxyglucose and annexin A5, which binds phosphatidyl serine, a thrombogenic lipid, on the cell membrane in macrophage-rich atherosclerotic lesions in mice [61]. Studies of human coronary arteries using ^{18}F-FDG-PET are limited due to cardiac ^{18}F-FDG uptake. A clinical study has demonstrated higher ^{18}F-FDG uptake in culprit lesions associated with acute coronary thrombosis compared with stable coronary lesions in patients with ischemic heart disease [62]. These lines of evidence might support the notion that arterial glucose uptake reflects plaque thrombogenicity and ^{18}F-FDG-PET is a minimally invasive method of detecting highly thrombogenic plaques.

5.2. Metabolism in atherosclerotic arteries

Cells uptake ^{18}F-FDG through glucose transporters and phosphorylate it by hexokinases. Thereafter, intracellular ^{18}F-FDG accumulates without further metabolism and is thus considered a marker of glucose utilization in tissues. Although systemic metabolic disorders such as dyslipidemia and diabetes accelerate the development of atherosclerosis, little is known about metabolic changes in atherosclerotic arteries and their significance in atherogenesis and

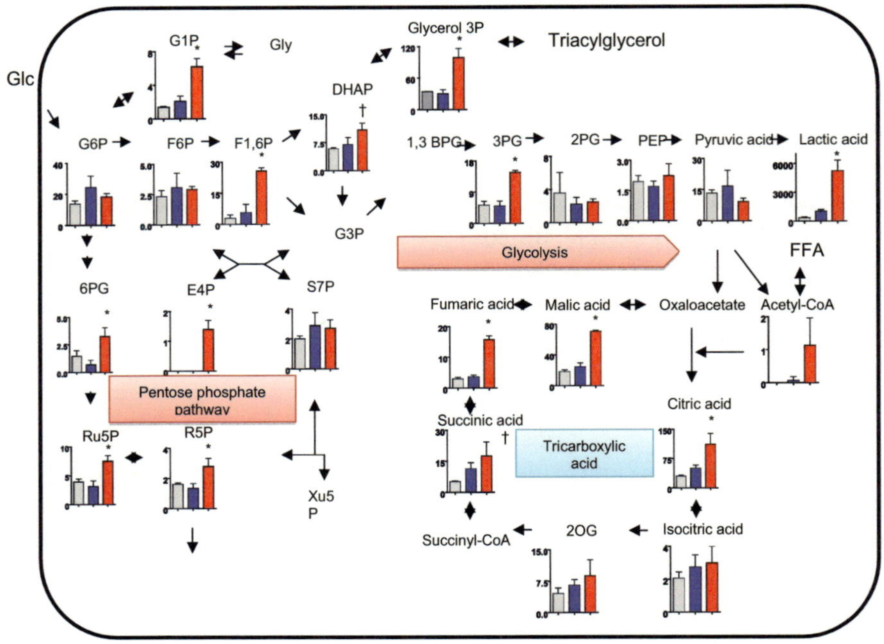

Figure 7. Levels of metabolites of glycolysis, the pentose phosphate pathway, tricarboxylic acid cycle, and glyconeogenesis/glycogenolysis in rabbit iliac–femoral arteries. Gray, blue, and red bars: iliac–femoral arteries that were not injured (conventional diet) and those with SMC-rich (conventional diet) and macrophage-rich (0.5% cholesterol diet) lesions, respectively ($n = 3$ for all). Metabolite levels are expressed as nanomole per gram; $^{*}p < 0.05$ vs. other groups, $^{\dagger}p < 0.05$ vs. noninjured femoral artery. Significant vascular metabolite changes in artery with macrophage-rich lesion. 1,3BPG, 1,3-bisphosphoglycerate; 2PG, 2-phosphoglyceric acid; 3PG, 3-phosphoglyceric acid; 2OG, 2-oxoglutaric acid; 6PG, 6-phosphogluconic acid; DHAP, dihydroxyacetone phosphate; E4P, erythrose 4-phosphate; F1-6P, fructose 1,6-diphosphate; F6P, fructose 6-phosphate; FFA, free fatty acid; G1P, glucose 1-phosphate; G3P, glyceraldehyde 3-phosphate; G6P, glucose 6-phosphate; Glu, glucose; Gly, glycogen; PEP, phosphoenolpyruvic acid; R5P, ribose 5-phosphate; Ru5P, ribulose 5-phosphate; S7P, sedoheptulose 7-phosphate; Xu5P, xylulose 5-phosphate (from Ref. 65).

thrombosis. Glucose utilization and O_2 consumption are increased in monkey and rabbit atherosclerotic aortic segments compared with nonatherosclerotic aortic segments [63]. In contrast, adenosine triphosphate (ATP) depletion in the cores of advanced atherosclerotic plaques is associated with hypoxic areas in the rabbit aorta [64]. We analyzed levels of central carbon metabolites in rabbit atherosclerotic arteries using capillary electrophoresis–time-of-flight mass spectrometry (CE-TOFMS) to determine comprehensive metabolic changes and hypoxic effects in atherosclerotic arteries. Macrophage-rich or SMC-rich lesions were generated by balloon injury in the iliac–femoral arteries of rabbits fed with a 0.5% cholesterol diet or a conventional diet. The number of proliferative cells increased in macrophage-rich arteries compared with control and SMC-rich arteries. Metabolites of glycolysis, the pentose phosphate pathway, the tricarboxylic acid cycle, and nucleotides increased in arteries with macrophage-rich lesions compared with noninjured control arteries and those with SMC-rich lesions [65] (Figure 7).

Hypoxic areas visualized by immunostaining pimonidazole hydrochloride were detectable only in arteries with macrophage-rich lesions, and they positively correlated with vascular

http://dx.doi.org/10.5772/61769

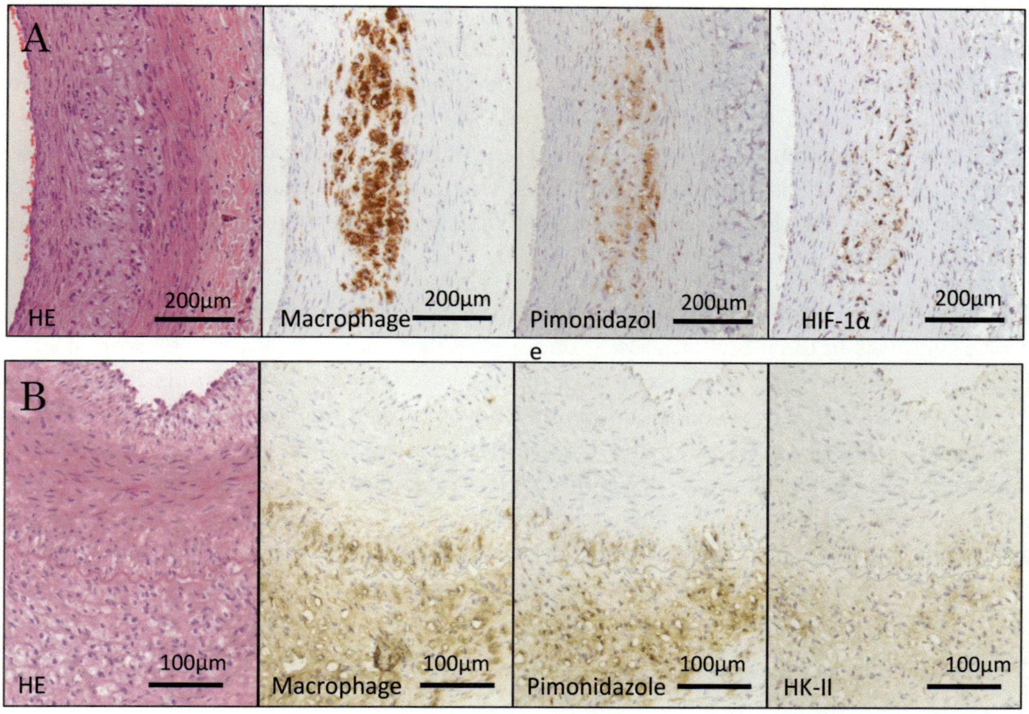

Figure 8. Immunohistochemical findings of hypoxia-inducible factor (HIF)-1α and hexokinase (HK)-II in iliac–femoral artery with macrophage-rich lesion. Immunohistochemical staining for macrophages, pimonidazole and HIF-1α in paraffin sections (A) and for macrophages, pimonidazole and HK-II in frozen sections (B). Nuclear translocation of HIF-1α and expression of HK-II in macrophage-rich hypoxic area. Hematoxylin eosin (HE stain) (from Ref. 65).

^{18}F-FDG uptake. The hypoxic areas were localized deep in the wall, and distributed in macrophage-rich areas with nuclear localization of hypoxia-inducible factor (HIF)-1α and hexokinase II expression [65] (Figure 8). Hypoxic responses might partly affect the glycolytic activity in macrophage-rich arteries. The cores of more advanced plaques > 500 μm thick were necrotic and hypoxic, and characterized by ATP depletion, low glucose and glycogen concentrations, and high lactate concentrations in the rabbit aorta [64]. The depletion of ATP might contribute to macrophage death and expansion of the necrotic core in atherosclerotic lesions. A hypoxic plaque has been detected in the rabbit atherosclerotic aorta using ^{18}F-fluoromisonidazole PET imaging [66]. Higher ^{18}F-fluoromisonidazole uptake by advanced atherosclerotic lesions is associated with hypoxic areas and neovascularization.

The pentose phosphate pathway is an alternative route for glucose catabolism that functions in the formation of ribose 5-phosphate (R5P) that is required for ribonucleic and deoxyribonucleic acid synthesis for cell growth and proliferation, and the formation of nicotinamide adenine dinucleotide phosphate (NADPH) for biosynthetic reactions. NADPH protects directly against oxidative stress by neutralizing reactive oxygen intermediates and indirectly via regenerating reduced glutathione. Studies have found both small and large amounts of metabolic flow through the pentose phosphate pathway in arteries compared with the glycolysis pathway [67, 68]. Increased amounts of metabolites of the pentose phosphate pathway are compatible with increased nucleotide levels and numbers of proliferative cells in macrophage-rich arteries [65]. The roles of the pentose phosphate pathway in atherosclerosis and atherothrombosis are poorly understood. A 20% reduction in normal levels of glucose 6-phosphate dehydrogenase activity, a key enzyme of pentose phosphate pathway, decreased serum cholesterol levels, vascular superoxide release, and atherosclerotic lesions but increased blood pressure in apoE-deficient mice suggest that this pathway exerts complex effects on atherogenesis [69].

The increase in glycerol 3-phosphate is compatible with increased phospholipid and triglyceride synthesis in the rabbit atherosclerotic aorta [70]. Atherosclerotic rabbits were injected with sodium acetate-1-C^{14} to assess its incorporation into arterial phospholipids. Radioactivity levels were higher in noncholine-containing phospholipids, phosphatidylcholine, sphingomyelin, and lysolecithin as well as triglycerides in atherosclerotic lesions than in corresponding plasma phospholipids, whereas $< 1\%$ of the label found in the phospholipids was incorporated into free cholesterol taken up by atherosclerotic lesions [70]. This suggests that phospholipids and triglycerides are synthesized in atherosclerotic lesions in situ, and that cholesterol is mainly derived from the plasma. These metabolic changes in atherosclerotic arteries could partly explain the metabolic changes in activated and/or hypoxic macrophages, as described below.

5.3. Metabolism of activated and/or hypoxic macrophages

Most cells produce ATP via glycolysis and oxidative phosphorylation under normoxic conditions, and mainly via glycolysis under hypoxic conditions. However, macrophages produce ATP via glycolysis even under normoxic conditions. The contributions of glucose, glutamine, and oleate to ATP production were measured in isolated mouse peritoneal macrophages using radiolabeled probes. The production of ATP in the macrophages was mediated by anaerobic glycolysis (54%), aerobic glutamine (24%), and fatty acid oxidation (22%) [71]. At an initial glucose concentration of 5 mM, almost all utilized glucose was converted into lactate through glycolysis, whereas only ~3% of glucose was oxidized under normoxic conditions [72]. The dependence of macrophages on glycolysis might be partly explained by the impaired HIF-1 inhibition. The cytoplasmic tail of the membrane type-1 matrix metalloprotease bound to factor inhibiting HIF-1 (FIH-1) leads to the inhibition of the FIH by the adaptor protein Mint3/APBA3 under normoxic conditions [73]. Because most of the genes related to glycolysis, such as those for glucose transporter 1, hexokinase, phosphofructokinase, phosphoglycerate kinase 1, are induced by HIF-1, the constitutive activation of HIF-1 might enhance the glycolysis pathway in normoxic macrophages. However, HIF-1α was translocated to the nucleus mainly in hypoxic areas but not in all macrophages in rabbit atherosclerotic lesions. Therefore, HIF-1-dependent and -independent pathways might contribute to the enhanced glycolytic pathway in macrophages in atherosclerotic lesions.

Macrophages comprise a heterogeneous cell population in terms of protein expression and function, both of which are affected by the microenvironment, and the metabolic status is also affected by macrophage activation pathways. Classical activation by lipopolysaccharide (LPS) and/or interferon-γ enhances the glycolysis pathway and lactate production, whereas an alternative pathway (interleukin-4 and -13) enhances fatty acid oxidation [74–76]. Hypoxia, but not pro-inflammatory cytokines, notably stimulates glucose uptake in human macrophages and foam cells, whereas pro-inflammatory cytokines stimulate glucose uptake in SMCs and endothelial cells [77]. We analyzed levels of 110 cationic and anionic metabolites in classically activated THP-1 macrophages under normoxic and hypoxic (1% O_2) conditions to determine comprehensive metabolic changes in macrophages. Under normoxic conditions, one-third of metabolite levels differed in the macrophages stimulated by lipopolysaccharides and interferon-γ, while metabolites of the glycolysis and pentose phosphate pathways did not increase in activated macrophages compared with nonstimulated macrophages. Hypoxia increased metabolite levels of glycolysis and the pentose phosphate pathway and decreased metabolite levels of tricarboxylic acid cycle in the activated macrophages. The results of a comprehensive metabolic analysis support the notion that hypoxia augments glucose utilization through the glycolysis and pentose phosphate pathways in classically activated macrophages [65]. This study suggested that metabolic changes occur in nucleotides, amino acids, and other charged metabolites in classically activated hypoxic macrophages.

Hypoxia also affects lipid metabolism in macrophages and foam cell formation. Increases of 50% and 120% in cholesterol and triglyceride contents, respectively, under hypoxic conditions (1% O_2), were accompanied by elevated 3-hydroxy-3-methyl-glutaryl-CoA reductase activities. Cholesterol-efflux assays showed that hypoxia significantly decreased the efflux mediated by the subcellular distribution of the ATP-binding cassette subfamily A member 1 (ABCA1). The hypoxia-induced accumulation of sterol and decreased cholesterol efflux was partly mediated by HIF-1α [78]. Other pathways might also contribute to the lipid metabolism in hypoxic macrophages. Cholesterol efflux mediated by ABCA1 is regulated by HIF-1β in primary human macrophages under hypoxia [79]. Positive interaction between liver X receptor α and HIF-1α synergistically induces triglyceride accumulation and foam cell formation in human primary macrophages and RAW 264.7 cells under hypoxia [80]. The expression of the secreted proteoglycan, versican, is enhanced in hypoxic macrophages, which might increase lipoprotein retention in microenvironments as well as the lipid content of hypoxic macrophages [81].

Changes in metabolism or in metabolites can alter the inflammatory response of activated macrophages. The heterozygous disruption of inducible 6-phosphofructo-2-kinase, a rate-limiting glycolysis enzyme, enhances pro-inflammatory gene expression in adipose tissue macrophages from mice fed with a high-fat diet [82]. A kinase screening has identified downregulation of sedoheptulose kinase, an enzyme of the pentose phosphate pathway, in LPS-stimulated RAW 264.7 macrophages. The reduction of sedoheptulose kinase in activated macrophages is associated with greater flux through glycolysis and the oxidative pentose phosphate pathway, which results in an increased overall redox potential and a reduced rate of O_2 consumption [83]. The overexpression of glucose-6-phosphate dehydrogenase, the first and rate-limiting enzyme of the pentose phosphate pathway, stimulates NF-κB transcriptional activity and promotes oxidative stress and inflammatory responses in RAW 264.7 macrophages [84]. These findings suggest cross talk between macrophage activation pathways and metabolism. With respect to atherogenesis, a deficiency of fatty acid synthase or a long-chain fatty acid elongase reduces atherosclerosis in apoE- or low-density receptor-deficient mice [85, 86].

5.4. Hypoxia links atherometabolism to vascular thrombogenicity

Arterial glucose uptake reflects vascular thrombogenicity in rabbits [60]. However, the underlying mechanisms remain unclear. Hypoxia is an important microenvironmental factor that influences the progression of atherosclerosis by inducing foam cell formation and necrotic core expansion, metabolic changes in infiltrative macrophages, and plaque neovascularization. Sluimer et al. [87] used the hypoxia marker pimonidazole hydrochloride to reveal hypoxic areas in the center of an advanced human carotid plaque and found that they correlated with the presence of thrombus, angiogenesis, microvessel density and the expression of hexokinase, HIF, and vascular endothelial growth factor. Hypoxia upregulates TF in the lungs [88], plasminogen activator inhibitor (PAI)-1 in hepatocytes [89], and ecto-nucleoside triphosphate diphosphohydrolase 1 (ecto-NTPDase 1) expression in endothelial cells [90]. TF and PAI-1 promote fibrin formation by initiating the coagulation cascade and inhibiting fibrinolysis, respectively, whereas ecto-NTPDase inhibits platelet aggregation via the hydrolysis of extracellular adenosine diphosphate. Because these three molecules are expressed in human atherosclerotic plaques [4, 91, 92], hypoxic conditions in the plaques can affect vascular thrombogenicity and arterial thrombus formation. We examined the effects of hypoxia in arterial thrombus formation using rabbit model of atherosclerosis, atherothrombosis, cultured macrophages, and human coronary plaques with or without acute coronary thrombosis. Atherosclerotic lesions were induced in rabbit femoral arteries by a 0.5%-cholesterol diet and balloon injury. Hypoxic areas detected by pimonidazole immunoreactivity were localized in the lipid and macrophage-rich deep portions of the plaque and a few superficial cells, but not in uninjured arteries. The extent of the hypoxic areas correlated with the plaque size, macrophage content, the nuclear localization of HIF-1α and NF-κB p65, and TF expression. Hypoxic areas in arteries closely correlated with fibrin areas in thrombus induced by a balloon catheter and hypoxia (1% O_2) enhanced the nuclear localization of HIF-1α and NF-κB p65, as well as TF expression and procoagulant activity in cultured macrophages [93]. The enhanced TF activity was suppressed by the inhibitors of either HIF-1 or NF-κB, suggesting that HIF-1 and NF-κB exert synergic effects upon procoagulant activities in hypoxic plaques [93]. These findings suggested that hypoxia promotes arterial fibrin formation via the augmentation of vascular thrombogenicity in rabbits. Coronary plaques contain more abundant macrophages, T lymphocytes, and fibrin deposition in patients with unstable angina pectoris than in patients with stable angina pectoris. The expression of TF, PAI-1, HIF-1α, and NF-κB p65 is closely distributed in coronary thrombotic plaques, and the nuclear localization of HIF-1α correlates with the expression of NF-κB p65, TF, PAI-1, and fibrin [93]. The pathological findings support the notion that hypoxic and nonhypoxic, possibly inflammatory, stimuli enhance thrombogenicity in symptomatic plaques. Because hypoxia enhances glucose uptake and glycolysis flux in atherosclerotic lesions and macrophages as described above, hypoxia might link glucose metabolism and thrombogenicity in atherosclerotic plaques.

http://dx.doi.org/10.5772/61769

6. Conclusion

The pathological findings suggest that the enhanced platelet aggregation and fibrin formation result in occlusive thrombus formation on disrupted atherosclerotic plaques. The size of the arterial thrombus would be affected by the degree of plaque disruption, the amount of exposed TF and platelet agonists, changes in blood flow, and the geographic features of disrupted plaques. Disrupted blood flow and excess thrombin generation can amplify blood coagulation and platelet recruitment to the thrombus surface and sustain platelet activation. Arterial glucose uptake reflects vascular thrombogenicity. These findings might be partly explained by metabolic adaptation and enhanced procoagulant activity under a hypoxic microenvironment, although further study is required. The relationship might provide new insight into novel therapeutic targets for atherothrombosis and the noninvasive detection of high-risk plaques.

Acknowledgements

The work was supported in part by Grants-in-Aid for Scientific Research in Japan (Nos. 25460440, 23390084) from the Ministry of Education, Science, Sports and Culture of Japan, Mitsui Life Welfare Foundation, an Intramural Research Fund (25-4-3) for Cardiovascular Diseases from the National Cerebral and Cardiovascular Center, and the Integrated Research Project for Human and Veterinary Medicine.

Author details

Atsushi Yamashita* and Yujiro Asada

*Address all correspondence to: atsushi_yamashita@med.miyazaki-u.ac.jp

University of Miyazaki, Miyazaki, Japan

References

[1] Sato Y, Hatakeyama K, Marutsuka K, Asada Y. Incidence of asymptomatic coronary thrombosis and plaque disruption: comparison of non-cardiac and cardiac deaths among autopsy cases. Thromb Res. 2009;124:19–23.

[2] Burke AP, Kolodgie FD, Farb A, Weber DK, Malcom GT, Smialek J, Virmani R. Healed plaque ruptures and sudden coronary death: evidence that subclinical rupture has a role in plaque progression. Circulation. 2001;103:934–40.

[3] Bentzon JF, Otsuka F, Virmani R, Falk E. Mechanisms of plaque formation and rupture. Circ Res. 2014;114:1852–66.

[4] Hatakeyama K, Asada Y, Marutsuka K, Sato Y, Kamikubo Y, Sumiyoshi A. Localization and activity of tissue factor in human aortic atherosclerotic lesions. Atherosclerosis. 1997;133:213–19.

[5] Oemar BS, Tschudi MR, Godoy N, Brovkovich V, Malinski T, Lüscher TF. Reduced endothelial nitric oxide synthase expression and production in human atherosclerosis. Circulation. 1998;97:2494–98.

[6] Monaco C, Andreakos E, Kiriakidis S, Mauri C, Bicknell C, Foxwell B, Cheshire N, Paleolog E, Feldmann M. Canonical pathway of nuclear factor kappa B activation selectively regulates proinflammatory and prothrombotic responses in human atherosclerosis. Proc Natl Acad Sci U S A. 2004;101:5634–39.

[7] Ogawa M, Ishino S, Mukai T, Asano D, Teramoto N, Watabe H, Kudomi N, Shiomi M, Magata Y, Iida H, Saji H. (18)F-FDG accumulation in atherosclerotic plaques: immunohistochemical and PET imaging study. J Nucl Med. 2004;45:1245–50.

[8] Tahara N, Kai H, Yamagishi S, Mizoguchi M, Nakaura H, Ishibashi M, Kaida H, Baba K, Hayabuchi N, Imaizumi T. Vascular inflammation evaluated by [18F]-fluorodeoxyglucose positron emission tomography is associated with the metabolic syndrome. J Am Coll Cardiol. 2007;49:1533–39.

[9] Rominger A, Saam T, Wolpers S, Cyran CC, Schmidt M, Foerster S, Nikolaou K, Reiser MF, Bartenstein P, Hacker M. 18F-FDG PET/CT identifies patients at risk for future vascular events in an otherwise asymptomatic cohort with neoplastic disease. J Nucl Med. 2009;50:1611–20.

[10] Aziz K, Berger K, Claycombe K, Huang R, Patel R, Abela GS. Noninvasive detection and localization of vulnerable plaque and arterial thrombosis with computed tomography angiography/positron emission tomography. Circulation. 2008;117:2061–70.

[11] Yamashita A, Sumi T, Goto S, Hoshiba Y, Nishihira K, Kawamoto R, Hatakeyama K, Date H, Imamura T, Ogawa H, Asada Y. Detection of von Willebrand factor and tissue factor in platelets-fibrin rich coronary thrombi in acute myocardial infarction. Am J Cardiol. 2006;97:26–28.

[12] Nishihira K, Yamashita A, Ishikawa T, Hatakeyama K, Shibata Y, Asada Y. Composition of thrombi in late drug-eluting stent thrombosis versus de novo acute myocardial infarction. Thromb Res. 2010;126:254–57.

[13] Rittersma SZ, van der Wal AC, Koch KT, Piek JJ, Henriques JP, Mulder KJ, Ploegmakers JP, Meesterman M, de Winter RJ. Plaque instability frequently occurs days or weeks before occlusive coronary thrombosis: a pathological thrombectomy study in primary percutaneous coronary intervention. Circulation. 2005;111:1160–65.

[14] Nishihira K, Hatakeyama K, Shibata Y, Kitamura K, Asada Y. Organized thrombus in aspirated coronary materials can predict in-hospital mortality of patients with acute myocardial infarction. Circ J. 2013;77:1275–80.

[15] Kramer MC, van der Wal AC, Koch KT, Ploegmakers JP, van der Schaaf RJ, Henriques JP, Baan J Jr, Rittersma SZ, Vis MM, Piek JJ, Tijssen JG, de Winter RJ. Presence of older thrombus is an independent predictor of long-term mortality in patients with ST-elevation myocardial infarction treated with thrombus aspiration during primary percutaneous coronary intervention. Circulation. 2008;118:1810–16.

[16] Virmani R, Kolodgie FD, Burke AP, Farb A, Schwartz SM. Lessons from sudden coronary death: a comprehensive morphological classification scheme for atherosclerotic lesions. Arterioscler Thromb Vasc Biol. 2000;20:1262–75.

[17] Kolodgie FD, Burke AP, Farb A, Gold HK, Yuan J, Narula J, Finn AV, Virmani R. The thin-cap fibroatheroma: a type of vulnerable plaque: the major precursor lesion to acute coronary syndromes. Curr Opin Cardiol. 2001;16:285–92.

[18] van der Wal AC, Becker AE, van der Loos CM, Das PK. Site of intimal rupture or erosion of thrombosed coronary atherosclerotic plaques is characterized by an inflammatory process irrespective of the dominant plaque morphology. Circulation. 1994;89:36–44.

[19] Sato Y, Hatakeyama K, Yamashita A, Marutsuka K, Sumiyoshi A, Asada Y. Proportion of fibrin and platelets differs in thrombi on ruptured and eroded coronary atherosclerotic plaques in humans. Heart. 2005;91:526–30.

[20] Okada K, Ueda Y, Matsuo K, Nishio M, Hirata A, Kashiwase K, Asai M, Nemoto T, Kodama K. Frequency and healing of nonculprit coronary artery plaque disruptions in patients with acute myocardial infarction. Am J Cardiol. 2011;107:1426–29.

[21] Davies MJ, Bland JM, Hangartner JR, Angelini A, Thomas AC. Factors influencing the presence or absence of acute coronary artery thrombi in sudden ischaemic death. Eur Heart J. 1989;10:203–08.

[22] Arbustini E, Grasso M, Diegoli M, Morbini P, Aguzzi A, Fasani R, Specchia G. Coronary thrombosis in non-cardiac death. Coron Artery Dis. 1993;4:751–59.

[23] Mauriello A, Servadei F, Sangiorgi G, Anemona L, Giacobbi E, Liotti D, Spagnoli LG. Asymptomatic carotid plaque rupture with unexpected thrombosis over a non-canonical vulnerable lesion. Atherosclerosis. 2011;218:356–62.

[24] Fry DL. Acute vascular endothelial changes associated with increased blood velocity gradients. Circ Res. 1968;22:165–97.

[25] Yamashita A, Asada Y, Sugimura H, Yamamoto H, Marutsuka K, Hatakeyama K, Tamura S, Ikeda Y, Sumiyoshi A. Contribution of von Willebrand factor to thrombus formation on neointima of rabbit stenotic iliac artery under high blood-flow velocity. Arterioscler Thromb Vasc Biol. 2003;23:1105–10.

[26] Sumi T, Yamashita A, Matsuda S, Goto S, Nishihira K, Furukoji E, Sugimura H, Kawahara H, Imamura T, Kitamura K, Tamura S, Asada Y. Disturbed blood flow induces erosive injury to smooth muscle cell-rich neointima and promotes thrombus formation in rabbit femoral artery. J Thromb Haemost. 2010;8:1394–402.

[27] Sameshima N, Yamashita A, Sato S, Matsuda S, Matsuura Y, Asada Y. The values of wall shear stress, turbulence kinetic energy and blood pressure gradient are associated with atherosclerotic plaque erosion in rabbits. J Atheroscler Thromb. 2014;21:831–38.

[28] Shiomi M, Ishida T, Kobayashi T, Nitta N, Sonoda A, Yamada S, Koike T, Kuniyoshi N, Murata K, Hirata K, Ito T, Libby P. Vasospasm of atherosclerotic coronary arteries precipitates acute ischemic myocardial damage in myocardial infarction-prone strain of the Watanabe heritable hyperlipidemic rabbits. Arterioscler Thromb Vasc Biol. 2013;33:2518–23.

[29] Miyamoto S, Ogawa H, Soejima H, Takazoe K, Kajiwara I, Shimomura H, Sakamoto T, Yoshimura M, Kugiyama K, Yasue H, Ozaki Y. Enhanced platelet aggregation in the coronary circulation after coronary spasm. Thromb Res. 2001;103:377–86.

[30] Oshima S, Yasue H, Ogawa H, Okumura K, Matsuyama K. Fibrinopeptide A is released into the coronary circulation after coronary spasm. Circulation. 1990;82:2222–25.

[31] Østerud, B. Tissue factor expression in blood cells. Thromb Res. 2010;125 Suppl 1:S31–S34.

[32] Mackman, N. Role of tissue factor in hemostasis, thrombosis, and vascular development. Arterioscler Thromb Vasc Biol. 2004;24:1015–22.

[33] Chou J, Mackman N, Merrill-Skoloff G, Pedersen B, Furie BC, Furie B. Hematopoietic cell-derived microparticle tissue factor contributes to fibrin formation during thrombus propagation. Blood. 2004;104:3190–97.

[34] Wang L, Miller C, Swarthout RF, Rao M, Mackman N, Taubman MB. Vascular smooth muscle-derived tissue factor is critical for arterial thrombosis after ferric chloride-induced injury. Blood. 2009;113:705–13.

[35] Yamashita A, Matsuda S, Matsumoto T, Moriguchi-Goto S, Takahashi M, Sugita C, Sumi T, Imamura T, Shima M, Kitamura K, Asada Y. Thrombin generation by intimal tissue factor contributes to thrombus formation on macrophage-rich neointima but not normal intima of hyperlipidemic rabbits. Atherosclerosis. 2009;206:418–26.

[36] Funatsu T, Yamashita A, Kaku S, Iwatsuki Y, Asada Y. Plasma factor Xa inhibition can predict antithrombotic effects of oral direct factor Xa inhibitors in rabbit atherothrombosis models. Thromb Haemost. 2012;108:896–902.

[37] Gailani D, Broze GJ Jr. Factor XI activation in a revised model of blood coagulation. Science. 1991;253:909–12.

[38] Yamashita A, Nishihira K, Kitazawa T, Yoshihashi K, Soeda T, Esaki K, Imamura T, Hattori K, Asada Y. Factor XI contributes to thrombus propagation on injured neointima of the rabbit iliac artery. J Thromb Haemost. 2006;4:1496–501.

[39] van Montfoort ML, Kuijpers MJ, Knaup VL, Bhanot S, Monia BP, Roelofs JJ, Heemskerk JW, Meijers JC. Factor XI regulates pathological thrombus formation on acutely ruptured atherosclerotic plaques. Arterioscler Thromb Vasc Biol. 2014;34:1668–73.

[40] Kuijpers MJ, van der Meijden PE, Feijge MA, Mattheij NJ, May F, Govers-Riemslag J, Meijers JC, Heemskerk JW, Renné T, Cosemans JM. Factor XII regulates the pathological process of thrombus formation on ruptured plaques. Arterioscler Thromb Vasc Biol. 2014;34:1674–80.

[41] Doggen CJ, Rosendaal FR, Meijers JC. Levels of intrinsic coagulation factors and the risk of myocardial infarction among men: opposite and synergistic effects of factors XI and XII. Blood. 2006;108:4045–51.

[42] Salomon O, Steinberg DM, Dardik R, Rosenberg N, Zivelin A, Tamarin I, Ravid B, Berliner S, Seligsohn U. Inherited factor XI deficiency confers no protection against acute myocardial infarction. J Thromb Haemost. 2003;1:658–61.

[43] Salomon O, Steinberg DM, Koren-Morag N, Tanne D, Seligsohn U. Reduced incidence of ischemic stroke in patients with severe factor XI deficiency. Blood. 2008;111:4113–17.

[44] Salomon O, Steinberg DM, Zucker M, Varon D, Zivelin A, Seligsohn U. Patients with severe factor XI deficiency have a reduced incidence of deep-vein thrombosis. Thromb Haemost. 2011;105:269-73. doi: 10.1160/TH10-05-0307.

[45] Kulkarni S, Dopheide SM, Yap CL, Ravanat C, Freund M, Mangin P, Heel KA, Street A, Harper IS, Lanza F, Jackson SP. A revised model of platelet aggregation. J Clin Invest. 2000;105:783–91.

[46] Bergmeier W, Piffath CL, Goerge T, Cifuni SM, Ruggeri ZM, Ware J, Wagner DD. The role of platelet adhesion receptor GPIbalpha far exceeds that of its main ligand, von Willebrand factor, in arterial thrombosis. Proc Natl Acad Sci U S A. 2006;103:16900–05.

[47] Yamashita A, Furukoji E, Marutsuka K, Hatakeyama K, Yamamoto H, Tamura S, Ikeda Y, Sumiyoshi A, Asada Y. Increased vascular wall thrombogenicity combined with reduced blood flow promotes occlusive thrombus formation in rabbit femoral artery. Arterioscler Thromb Vasc Biol. 2004;24:2420–24.

[48] Nesbitt WS, Giuliano S, Kulkarni S, Dopheide SM, Harper IS, Jackson SP. Intercellular calcium communication regulates platelet aggregation and thrombus growth. J Cell Biol. 2003;160:1151–61.

[49] Goto S, Tamura N, Ishida H, Ruggeri ZM. Dependence of platelet thrombus stability on sustained glycoprotein IIb/IIIa activation through adenosine 5'-diphosphate receptor stimulation and cyclic calcium signaling. J Am Coll Cardiol. 2006;47:155–62.

[50] Marzilli M, Sambuceti G, Fedele S, L'Abbate A. Coronary microcirculatory vasoconstriction during ischemia in patients with unstable angina. J Am Coll Cardiol. 2000;35:327–34.

[51] Schwartz RS, Burke A, Farb A, Kaye D, Lesser JR, Henry TD, Virmani R. Microemboli and microvascular obstruction in acute coronary thrombosis and sudden coronary death: relation to epicardial plaque histopathology. J Am Coll Cardiol. 2009;54:2167–73.

[52] Nishihira K, Yamashita A, Tanaka N, Kawamoto R, Imamura T, Yamamoto R, Eto T, Asada Y. Inhibition of 5-hydroxytryptamine receptor prevents occlusive thrombus formation on neointima of the rabbit femoral artery. J Thromb Haemost. 2006;4:247–55.

[53] Nishihira K, Yamashita A, Tanaka N, Moriguchi-Goto S, Imamura T, Ishida T, Kawashima S, Yamamoto R, Kitamura K, Asada Y. Serotonin induces vasoconstriction of smooth muscle cell-rich neointima through 5-hydroxytryptamine2A receptor in rabbit femoral arteries. J Thromb Haemost. 2008;6:1207–14.

[54] Nesbitt WS, Westein E, Tovar-Lopez FJ, Tolouei E, Mitchell A, Fu J, Carberry J, Fouras A, Jackson SP. A shear gradient-dependent platelet aggregation mechanism drives thrombus formation. Nat Med. 2009;15:665–73.

[55] Siedlecki CA, Lestini BJ, Kottke-Marchant KK, Eppell SJ, Wilson DL, Marchant RE. Shear-dependent changes in the three-dimensional structure of human von Willebrand factor. Blood. 1996;88:2939–50.

[56] Ikeda Y, Handa M, Kawano K, Kamata T, Murata M, Araki Y, Anbo H, Kawai Y, Watanabe K, Itagaki I. The role of von Willebrand factor and fibrinogen in platelet aggregation under varying shear stress. J Clin Invest. 1991;87:1234–40.

[57] Moreno-Sánchez R, Rodríguez-Enríquez S, Marín-Hernández A, Saavedra E. Energy metabolism in tumor cells. FEBS J. 2007;274:1393–418.

[58] Ghesquière B, Wong BW, Kuchnio A, Carmeliet P. Metabolism of stromal and immune cells in health and disease. Nature. 2014;511:167–76.

[59] Grandpierre S, Desandes E, Meneroux B, Djaballah W, Mandry D, Netter F, Wahl D, Fay R, Karcher G, Marie PY. Arterial foci of F-18 fluorodeoxyglucose are associated with an enhanced risk of subsequent ischemic stroke in cancer patients: a case-control pilot study. Clin Nucl Med. 2011;36:85–90.

[60] Yamashita A, Zhao Y, Zhao S, Matsuura Y, Sugita C, Iwakiri T, Okuyama N, Ohe K, Koshimoto C, Kawai K, Tamaki N, Kuge Y, Asada Y. Arterial (18)F-fluorodeoxyglucose uptake reflects balloon catheter-induced thrombus formation and tissue factor

expression via nuclear factor-κB in rabbit atherosclerotic lesions. Circ J. 2013;77:2626–35.

[61] Zhao Y, Zhao S, Kuge Y, Strauss WH, Blankenberg FG, Tamaki N. Localization of deoxyglucose and annexin A5 in experimental atheroma correlates with macrophage infiltration but not lipid deposition in the lesion. Mol Imaging Biol. 2011;13:712–20.

[62] Rogers IS, Nasir K, Figueroa AL, Cury RC, Hoffmann U, Vermylen DA, Brady TJ, Tawakol A. Feasibility of FDG imaging of the coronary arteries: comparison between acute coronary syndrome and stable angina. JACC Cardiovasc Imaging. 2010;3:388–97.

[63] Morrison ES, Scott RF, Kroms M, Frick J. Glucose degradation in normal and atherosclerotic aortic intima-media. Atherosclerosis. 1972;16:175–84.

[64] Leppänen O, Björnheden T, Evaldsson M, Borén J, Wiklund O, Levin M. ATP depletion in macrophages in the core of advanced rabbit atherosclerotic plaques in vivo. Atherosclerosis. 2006;188:323–30.

[65] Yamashita A, Zhao Y, Matsuura Y, Yamasaki K, Moriguchi-Goto S, Sugita C, Iwakiri T, Okuyama N, Koshimoto C, Kawai K, Tamaki N, Zhao S, Kuge Y, Asada Y. Increased metabolite levels of glycolysis and pentose phosphate pathway in rabbit atherosclerotic arteries and hypoxic macrophage. PLoS One. 2014;9:e86426.

[66] Mateo J, Izquierdo-Garcia D, Badimon JJ, Fayad ZA, Fuster V. Noninvasive assessment of hypoxia in rabbit advanced atherosclerosis using ^{18}F-fluoromisonidazole positron emission tomographic imaging. Circ Cardiovasc Imaging. 2014;7:312–20.

[67] Lofland HB Jr, Moury DM, Hoffman CW, Clarkson TB. Lipid metabolism in pigeon aorta during atherogenesis. J Lipid Res. 1965;6:112–18.

[68] Whereat AF. Recent advances in experimental and molecular pathology. Atherosclerosis and metabolic disorder in the arterial wall. Exp Mol Pathol. 1967;7:233–47.

[69] Matsui R, Xu S, Maitland KA, Mastroianni R, Leopold JA, Handy DE, Loscalzo J, Cohen RA. Glucose-6-phosphate dehydrogenase deficiency decreases vascular superoxide and atherosclerotic lesions in apolipoprotein E(-/-) mice. Arterioscler Thromb Vasc Biol. 2006;26:910–16.

[70] Newman HA, McCandless EL, Zilversmit DB. The synthesis of C14-lipids in rabbit atheromatous lesions. J Biol Chem. 1961;236:1264–68.

[71] Newsholme P, Newsholme EA. Rates of utilization of glucose, glutamine and oleate and formation of end-products by mouse peritoneal macrophages in culture. Biochem J. 1989;261:211–18.

[72] Newsholme P, Gordon S, Newsholme EA. Rates of utilization and fates of glucose, glutamine, pyruvate, fatty acids and ketone bodies by mouse macrophages. Biochem J. 1987;242:631–36.

[73] Sakamoto T1, Seiki M. A membrane protease regulates energy production in macrophages by activating hypoxia-inducible factor-1 via a non-proteolytic mechanism. J Biol Chem. 2010;285:29951–64.

[74] Vats D, Mukundan L, Odegaard JI, Zhang L, Smith KL, Morel CR, Wagner RA, Greaves DR, Murray PJ, Chawla A. Oxidative metabolism and PGC-1beta attenuate macrophage-mediated inflammation. Cell Metab. 2006;4:13–24.

[75] Satomi T, Ogawa M, Mori I, Ishino S, Kubo K, Magata Y, Nishimoto T. Comparison of contrast agents for atherosclerosis imaging using cultured macrophages: FDG versus ultrasmall superparamagnetic iron oxide. J Nucl Med. 2013;54:999–1004.

[76] Tavakoli S, Zamora D, Ullevig S, Asmis R. Bioenergetic profiles diverge during macrophage polarization: implications for the interpretation of 18F-FDG PET imaging of atherosclerosis. J Nucl Med. 2013;54:1661–67.

[77] Folco EJ, Sheikine Y, Rocha VZ, Christen T, Shvartz E, Sukhova GK, Di Carli MF, Libby P. Hypoxia but not inflammation augments glucose uptake in human macrophages: implications for imaging atherosclerosis with 18fluorine-labeled 2-deoxy-D-glucose positron emission tomography. J Am Coll Cardiol. 2011;58:603–14.

[78] Parathath S, Mick SL, Feig JE, Joaquin V, Grauer L, Habiel DM, Gassmann M, Gardner LB, Fisher EA. Hypoxia is present in murine atherosclerotic plaques and has multiple adverse effects on macrophage lipid metabolism. Circ Res. 2011;109:1141–52.

[79] Ugocsai P, Hohenstatt A, Paragh G, Liebisch G, Langmann T, Wolf Z, Weiss T, Groitl P, Dobner T, Kasprzak P, Göbölös L, Falkert A, Seelbach-Goebel B, Gellhaus A, Winterhager E, Schmidt M, Semenza GL, Schmitz G. HIF-1beta determines ABCA1 expression under hypoxia in human macrophages. Int J Biochem Cell Biol. 2010;42:241–52.

[80] Na TY, Lee HJ, Oh HJ, Huh S, Lee IK, Lee MO. Positive cross-talk between hypoxia inducible factor-1α and liver X receptor α induces formation of triglyceride-loaded foam cells. Arterioscler Thromb Vasc Biol. 2011;31:2949–56.

[81] Asplund A, Stillemark-Billton P, Larsson E, Rydberg EK, Moses J, Hultén LM, Fagerberg B, Camejo G, Bondjers G. Hypoxic regulation of secreted proteoglycans in macrophages. Glycobiology. 2010;20:33–40.

[82] Huo Y, Guo X, Li H, Wang H, Zhang W, Wang Y, Zhou H, Gao Z, Telang S, Chesney J, Chen YE, Ye J, Chapkin RS, Wu C. Disruption of inducible 6-phosphofructo-2-kinase ameliorates diet-induced adiposity but exacerbates systemic insulin resistance and adipose tissue inflammatory response. J Biol Chem. 2010;285:3713–21.

[83] Haschemi A, Kosma P, Gille L, Evans CR, Burant CF, Starkl P, Knapp B, Haas R, Schmid JA, Jandl C, Amir S, Lubec G, Park J, Esterbauer H, Bilban M, Brizuela L, Pospisilik JA, Otterbein LE, Wagner O. The sedoheptulose kinase CARKL directs macro-

phage polarization through control of glucose metabolism. Cell Metab. 2012;15:813–26.

[84] Ham M, Lee JW, Choi AH, Jang H, Choi G, Park J, Kozuka C, Sears DD, Masuzaki H, Kim JB. Macrophage glucose-6-phosphate dehydrogenase stimulates proinflammatory responses with oxidative stress. Mol Cell Biol. 2013;33:2425–35.

[85] Schneider JG, Yang Z, Chakravarthy MV, Lodhi IJ, Wei X, Turk J, Semenkovich CF. Macrophage fatty-acid synthase deficiency decreases diet-induced atherosclerosis. J Biol Chem. 2010;285:23398–409.

[86] Saito R, Matsuzaka T, Karasawa T, Sekiya M, Okada N, Igarashi M, Matsumori R, Ishii K, Nakagawa Y, Iwasaki H, Kobayashi K, Yatoh S, Takahashi A, Sone H, Suzuki H, Yahagi N, Yamada N, Shimano H. Macrophage Elovl6 deficiency ameliorates foam cell formation and reduces atherosclerosis in low-density lipoprotein receptor-deficient mice. Arterioscler Thromb Vasc Biol. 2011;31:1973–79.

[87] Sluimer JC, Gasc JM, van Wanroij JL, Kisters N, Groeneweg M, Sollewijn Gelpke MD, Cleutjens JP, van den Akker LH, Corvol P, Wouters BG, Daemen MJ, Bijnens AP. Hypoxia, hypoxia-inducible transcription factor, and macrophages in human atherosclerotic plaques are correlated with intraplaque angiogenesis. J Am Coll Cardiol. 2008;51:1258–65.

[88] Yan SF, Zou YS, Gao Y, Zhai C, Mackman N, Lee SL, Milbrandt J, Pinsky D, Kisiel W, Stern D. Tissue factor transcription driven by Egr-1 is a critical mechanism of murine pulmonary fibrin deposition in hypoxia. Proc Natl Acad Sci U S A. 1998;95:8298–303.

[89] Kietzmann T, Roth U, Jungermann K. Induction of the plasminogen activator inhibitor-1 gene expression by mild hypoxia via a hypoxia response element binding the hypoxia-inducible factor-1 in rat hepatocytes. Blood. 1999;94:4177–85.

[90] Eltzschig HK, Köhler D, Eckle T, Kong T, Robson SC, Colgan SP. Central role of Sp1-regulated CD39 in hypoxia/ischemia protection. Blood. 2009;113:224–32.

[91] Hatakeyama K, Hao H, Imamura T, Ishikawa T, Shibata Y, Fujimura Y, Eto T, Asada Y. Relation of CD39 to plaque instability and thrombus formation in directional atherectomy specimens from patients with stable and unstable angina pectoris. Am J Cardiol. 2005;95:632–35.

[92] Raghunath PN, Tomaszewski JE, Brady ST, Caron RJ, Okada SS, Barnathan ES. Plasminogen activator system in human coronary atherosclerosis. Arterioscler Thromb Vasc Biol. 1995;15:1432–43.

[93] Matsuura Y, Yamashita A, Iwakiri T, Sugita C, Okuyama N, Kitamura K, Asada Y. Vascular wall hypoxia promotes arterial thrombus formation via augmentation of vascular thrombogenicity. Thromb Haemost. 2015; 114:158–72.

Chapter 2

NF-κB — A Key Factor in Atherogenesis and Atheroprogression

Francesca Bonomini, Gaia Favero and Rita Rezzani

Additional information is available at the end of the chapter

http://dx.doi.org/10.5772/61894

Abstract

Atherosclerosis is the major cause of cardiovascular diseases and it is responsible for a large proportion of mortality in the Western society.

Initially, atherosclerosis was thought to be a degenerative disease that was an inevitable consequence of aging. The recent research has shown that atherosclerosis is a slowly progressing inflammatory disease of the medium- and large-sized arteries, resulting in the formation of fatty and fibrous lesions.

Inflammatory processes mark all stages of atherogenesis: from early endothelial activation by modified lipids to eventual rupture of the atherosclerotic plaque. The inflammation of the vessel wall is a feature of this pathology, which is characterized by infiltration and oxidation of low-density lipoproteins (LDLs), increase in oxidative stress, with the consequent lipid accumulation in the vessel wall, and foam cells formation.

The extensive relation between the immune system and vessels induce the infiltration of immune cells into the vascular wall, the major pathogenic step in atherogenesis. At this aim, reactive oxygen species play a crucial role activating a number of redox-sensitive transcriptional factors such as nuclear factor kappa B (NF-κB), which is involved in transcription of many genes with an established role in atherosclerosis, such as cytokines, chemokines, adhesion molecules, acute phase proteins, regulators of apoptosis, and cell proliferation. Since its discovery in 1986, the transcription factor NF-κB has evoked large attention on the basis of its peculiar regulation, the abundance of activation stimuli, the different genes and biological responses controlled, the striking evolutionary conservation of structure and function among family members, and its role in different human diseases.

Recognition of the leading role of inflammation at all stages of pathogenesis focuses on the potential relationship between systemic inflammation and atherosclerosis and fuelled intense basic science, health, and clinical research.

The understanding of the inflammation involvement in atherogenesis, atheroprogression, and its complications confirm the importance of traditional risk factors in this disease, such as high LDL levels. Indeed, inflammatory process can be considered a pathway that, from mechanistic and functional points of view, suggests a connection with the known risk factors and alterations to the vessel biology that drive to atheroprogression and its complications.

In this review, we discuss the transcription factor NF-κB and its potential role in atherogenesis and atheroprogression focusing on the major atherosclerotic factors regulated by NF-κB and how they may affect different steps in the atherosclerotic process.

Keywords: NF-κB, atherosclerosis, vessels

1. Introduction

Atherosclerosis is a disease of arteries with slow progression which induces the formation of lesions characterized by the accumulation of fatty and fibrous tissue in the vessel wall. It is one of the most important factor responsible for the mortality by cardiovascular diseases in developed countries, despite changes in lifestyle and the use of preventative pharmacological approaches. In the past years, after the understanding of the involvement of inflammation and immune response in the pathogenesis, atherosclerosis has been redefined as an inflammatory disease [1, 2].

The development of atherosclerotic lesions can be subdivided into initiation and expansion of fatty streaks. In the first step, activated vascular endothelium expresses inducible leukocyte adhesion molecules and chemokines. Once blood circulating leukocytes, in particular monocytes, adhere and enter into the artery wall, the cells differentiate into macrophages and, after lipidic phagocytosis, into foam cells. The macrophage and T-cell infiltration is a feature of the atherogenesis initiation called "fatty streaks formation" [3, 4].

After this step, there is production of cytokines and growth factors within lesions that may amplify monocyte recruitment, stimulate macrophage proliferation, and induce migration of smooth muscle cells into the intimal layer of the vessel, with consequent extracellular matrix proliferation and deposition, and "mature" plaques formation. This step of the atherosclerotic lesion is featured by the arrangement of a fibrous cap covering the lesion inside the internal elastic lamina constituted by fibrous tissue, with or without a lipidic core with foam cells and extracellular lipid deposits, determining a variable reduction of vascular lumen space [3].

Though clinically significant complications of atherosclerosis, such as plaque ulceration, rupture, and thrombosis, occur in established or advanced atherosclerotic plaques, understanding the mechanisms of lesion formation offers the possibility of intervening to delay or prevent lesion progression and complications.

Numerous transcription factors may be critical in both the initiation and the expansion of lesions, as well as in protecting the vessel wall from the formation of atherosclerotic lesions. In this summary, we focus our attention on one transcription factor, nuclear factor-κB (NF-κB), which is considered to be a major transcription factor regulating many functions of the vessel wall.

http://dx.doi.org/10.5772/61894

In the context of the multifactor pathogenesis of atherosclerosis, different stimuli have the possibility to activate NF-κB, comprising local factors such as vascular injury, as well as modified low-density lipoproteins (LDLs), infectious agents, and cytokines, although it is not easy to determine which of them are responsible for the activation of NF-κB in vivo. Indeed, NF-κB, throughout the lifetime of an individual, may be a convergence point integrating these different stimuli [3, 5].

2. Atherosclerotic pathogenic process

The atherosclerotic pathogenic process is initiated early in life, during postnatal development and maturation and advances gradually throughout life [6]. Given the multifactorial and complex nature of atherosclerosis, further studies to clarify the understanding of the pathogenic process are needed to improve atherosclerosis diagnosis, management, prevention, and treatment [7]. The first step in the atherosclerotic lesion formation is endothelial activation or dysfunction and LDL-cholesterol deposition in the arterial wall, which are mediated by risk factors such as dyslipidemia, hypertension, diabetes mellitus, and smoking. After this step, the accumulated LDLs are oxidized and the resultant formation of oxidized LDLs (OxLDLs) has been suggested to be the critical event in deteriorating inflammation in vascular wall. After this, not only monocytes but also various types of leukocytes adhere to the activated endothelium, migrate into the arterial wall via upregulated adhesion molecules, and produce pro-inflammatory cytokines or chemokines. Subsequently, monocyte-derived macrophages take up OxLDLs via scavenger receptor, leading to the formation of lipid-laden foam cells. Following such steps, the initial fatty streaks contain lipids and numerous immune cells such as macrophages, dendritic cells (DCs), and T lymphocytes. After these phases progressed, atherosclerotic lesions involve the migrated smooth muscle cells, debris, apoptotic cells, and extracellular matrix such as collagen and proteoglycans [8]. Finally, such indolent progressed atherosclerotic plaques may suddenly rupture and induce life-threatening thrombosis. The notable features of unstable rupture-prone plaque are infiltration of many inflammatory cells, large lipid core, and thin fibrous cap [9–11].

3. NF-κB

The eukaryotic family of NF-κB transcription factors are involved in the expression of over 150 genes that regulate a variety of cellular processes [12,13, 14].

In this family there are p50, p52, p65 (RelA), c-Rel, and RelB, that form various homo- and hetero-dimers, where the most common active form is the p50/RelA or p52/RelA heterodimer. NF-κB subunits dimerization produces complexes with different DNA-binding specificities and transactivation potential [14, 15, 16]. The N-terminal region of each member of the NF-κB family is conserved and is called Rel-homology domain, which contains the dimerization, nuclear localization, and DNA-binding domains [14, 15, 17]. Most cell types show inactive form of NF-κB complexes in the cytoplasm bound to inhibitory proteins known as IκBs and activated, by phosphorylation on conserved serine residues in the N-terminal portion of IκB, in response to multiple stimuli, including cytokines, infectious agents, and stress-inducing factors; this modification occurs at Ser-32 and Ser-36 in the case of IκBα [14, 18–21]. The degradation of the inhibitory subunit by the 26S proteasome by phosphorylation targets IκBα for ubiquitination by the Skp1/Cul-1/F-box ubiquitin ligase complex, which recognizes phosphorylated substrates, [14, 22, 23] activates NF-κB that translocates to the nucleus where it binds to its DNA-binding site (5'-GGGRNNYYCC-3') in the promoter or enhancer regions of specific genes. This activation is the last phase in the signal transduction pathway conducing from the cell surface to the nucleus. Phosphorylation of IκBs is a key event in the activation of NF-κB mediated by a multimeric complex, named as the IκB kinase (IKK) complex [14].

NF-κB is peculiar for the characteristic to have a rapid activation and downregulation; the activation of this factor induces IκBα, permitting switching off of the system and for this reason NF-κB activation, in physiological conditions, is a transitory phenomenon, which induces a right expression of immune and "stress" genes. On the contrary, in diseases such as rheumatoid arthritis, asthma, or inflammatory bowel disease, there is a prolonged or inappropriate activation of the NF-κB pathway and this dysregulation induces the enhanced inflammatory response, feature of these pathologic conditions. NF-κB is also considered as an important key factor in the development and progression of cardiovascular diseases, such as atherosclerosis and acute coronary syndromes [3].

4. NF-κB in atherosclerosis

In humans, atherosclerotic plaques have been identified as the activated NF-κB form that is not detected in normal vessels [14, 24]. In atherosclerotic environment, there are different factors that induce the NF-κB activation in vitro. Furthermore, increased expression of numerous genes important in early atherosclerotic lesion formation is known to be regulated by NF-κB [14, 25]. NF-κB activation regulates the expression of some molecules that are involved in recruiting circulating mononuclear leukocytes to the arterial intima, an important step in atherosclerosis, like vascular cell adhesion molecule 1 (VCAM-1), intercellular adhesion molecule 1 (ICAM-1), and E-selectin, and chemokines interleukin 8 (IL-8) and monocyte chemoattractant protein 1 (MCP-1), [14, 26–28]. The activated NF-κB was detected in different areas of human atherosclerotic lesion and, also, in intimal cells found in coronary arteries of pigs placed on a hypercholesterolemic diet [14, 29, 30].

NF-κB is activated in intima and media tunica in models of arterial injury; moreover, animals treated with a statin, 3-hydroxy-3-methylglutaryl (HMG)-Co-A reductase inhibitor, demonstrated a greater decrease of NF-κB activity in circulating mononuclear cells and reduction in the extent of atherosclerosis. All these observations suggest an involvement of NF-κB activation in atherosclerotic pathology [14, 31].

http://dx.doi.org/10.5772/61894

5. NF-κB in early stages of atherosclerosis

The endothelium, thanks to its strategic position between the plasma and the underlying vascular tissue and its constitutive properties, has extensive biological activities that have key importance for body homeostasis [32, 33]. Endothelial cells (EC) regulate the transport of plasma molecules, in physiological conditions, by receptor-mediated and receptor-independent transcytosis and endocytosis; this traffic is bidirectional to monitor vascular tone and to synthesize and secrete a large variety of factors. Moreover, the endothelial layer has an important role in the regulation of hemostasis, inflammation, immunity, signal transduction, and lipidic homeostasis [32, 34, 35]. Under pathological conditions such as hyperlipidaemia and/or hyperglycemia, alterations in endothelial function precede the development of atherosclerotic plaques and contribute decisively to their perpetuation and to the clinical manifestations of vascular diseases [32]. Multiple upstream pathways might be responsible for activating NF-κB in endothelial cells promoting the development of atherosclerosis. Supporting the critical role of NF-κB in inflammation-dependent endothelial dysfunction is evidence that pharmacological inhibition of NF-κB signaling significantly reduces cytokines and enhances endothelial-dependent dilation in old mice and humans [36–38].

The demonstration of the role of inflammation in endothelial dysfunction is produced by researches in which exogenous administration of pro-inflammatory cytokines was shown to produce endothelial dysfunction or endothelial activation in endothelial cells or isolated arterial vessels [39–42]. The activation of NF-κB in endothelial cells, event involved in atherogenesis, is due to multiple upstream pathways. Previous studies have provided compelling evidence that inhibition of MyD88-dependent signaling downstream of Toll-like receptors (TLR) 2 and 4 led to a reduction in atherosclerosis through a decrease in chemokine levels and macrophage recruitment [43, 44]; other works suggested that the function in atherogenesis of TLR4 is induced by endogenous ligands and not by bacterial products, because CD14 deficiency did not have a protective effect. The expression of TLR2 was shown to be increased in intimal layer of vessel areas with disturbed blood flow, and the lack of TLR2 has a protective effect in vessels of hypercholesterolemic mice lacking the low-density lipoprotein receptor (LDL-R) [43, 45]. Several other studies suggested that activation of TLR pathways by oxidized LDL could contribute to the expression of proinflammatory mediators and plaque development in atherosclerotic lesions [46, 47]. Activation of TLR on vascular endothelial cells by oxidized LDL, inducing activation of NF-κB and proinflammatory cytokine and adhesion molecules synthesis by the intima tunica predisposing vessels to atherosclerotic disease, through the experiments directed to investigating the role of TLR signaling in atherosclerosis were performed using animal models [43, 44, 45, 48], but they could not clearly indicate the cellular specificity of TLR responses. Studies employing endothelial TLR signaling manipulation will provide important insights to approach in atherosclerosis about a specific role of endothelial cells for TLR-induced responses. NF-κB activation in lesion-prone sites of vessels could be also induced by fluid mechanical forces by integrin signaling [43, 49, 50], suggesting that NF-κB activation may function during the very early stages of atherogenesis by promoting monocyte recruitment and plaque formation in areas of disturbed blood flow [43, 48]. In addition to exacerbating inflammation downstream of NF-κB transcription of pro-inflammatory cytokines, inflammatory signaling also stimulates O2− production and oxidative stress (and vice versa) through a number of mechanisms. These include increased NF-κB-mediated transcription of redox-sensitive genes like those encoding subunits of NADPH oxidase [51–53] that increase reactive oxygen species (ROS) bioavailability and further activation of IKK-NF-κB signaling. Thus, NF-κB lies at the center of a vicious cycle that can exacerbate oxidative stress and inflammation. Interestingly, endothelial NF-κB can impact the healthspan/lifespan beyond its effects on vascular function per se [42].

Indeed, recent researches showed that inhibition of endothelial cell-specific inhibition of NF-κB resulted in reduced development of atherosclerosis in vivo in atherosclerotic mouse models. These studies showed much evidence pointing the protective role of NF-κB signaling inhibition, in particular in endothelial cells, in atherosclerosis mouse models it has an athero-protective effect relevant to human disease. The specific NF-κB inhibition in endothelial cell induces a reduction in expression of adhesion molecules and other inflammatory mediators in vessel wall, so it prevents the recruitment of monocytes/macrophages into the first steps of atherosclerosis, resulting in disease prevention [43].

In atherogenesis, monocytes differentiate into macrophages, a protective event meant to eliminate accumulated, inflammatory components (i.e., oxidized LDL, oxLDL). Cholesterol is transported in the circulation by plasma lipoproteins, in particular, LDLs act as an exogeneous source of cholesterol and other cellular nutrients for various tissues, including the hepatic ones, where it is taken up through endocytosis. Another possibility is that LDLs may be caught extracellularly in vessels, where they are subjected to an environment favorable to various enzymatic and chemical modifications. The generation of bioactive lipid peroxidative products occurs in early stages of arterial lipoprotein modification without change in cellular receptor recognition of the particles.

Cell surface receptors for LDL (LDL-R) as well as scavenger receptors for modified LDL (SR-A, CD36, CD68) are expressed in monocyte-derived macrophages in arteries. While LDL particles with a minimal level of oxidation carry bioactive molecules, they are physically indistinguishable from native plasma LDL [54]. Cellular signals that induce the generation of oxidized lipids are not determined, but after the oxidation the LDL can be phagocytosed by macrophages through the scavenger receptors on the cell surfaces. The macrophages perform an important protective function by removing of oxidized LDLs, so the effects of modified LDLs on endothelial cells and smooth muscle cells are reduced. The ingestion of oxidized LDL leads to the accumulation of lipid peroxides and to the store of the excess cholesterol as cholesteryl esters within the cytoplasm, resulting in the formation of foam cells. Some evidences suggest that elevated levels of LDLs, in both native and oxidized form, modulate vascular cell gene expression acting as pro-oxidant signals. The exposure of monocytes to oxidized LDL for short time activates NF-κB and upregulates the expression of target genes, while their longer exposure can downregulate these responses [55]. The native form of LDLs and minimally oxidized LDLs induce endothelial cells production of different NF-κB-dependent chemokines and adhesion molecules and, at the same time, components of oxidized LDL, such as lysophosphatidylcholine, induce expression of mononuclear leukocyte adhesion molecules and can activate NF-κB in the same cells [56, 57]. Production of these chemokines may amplify inflammation through the stimulation of resident macrophages proliferation and the recruitment of new monocytes into lesion sites. Moreover, pro-inflammatory cytokines expression in lesions can induce an increase in LDL binding to endothelium and smooth muscle cells and upregulates the expression of the LDL receptor, leading to further inflammation [24].

For the study of LDL, local oxidation, and its effects in arterial wall, Calara et al. [58] injected human LDL particles into a rat model and showed that these lipoproteins underwent oxidative modification with an activation of the endothelial NF-κB pathway and expression of NF-κB-dependent genes [58]. Other studies demonstrated arterial activation of NF-κB by very low-density lipoprotein (VLDL) and the consequent increased expression of NF-κB-dependent genes [59]. All these studies suggest that both LDL and VLDL may induce atherosclerosis in vessels of animal models involving NF-κB activation [24].

Atherosclerotic lesion is characterized by the migration of muscle cells from the tunica media to the tunica intima and their proliferation [3]. Moreover, smooth muscle cell proliferation, termed "neointimal hyperplasia", after percutaneous interventions is a trademark of restenosis [3]. Because vascular injury is the major stimulus for NF-κB activation and smooth muscle cell proliferation, as described earlier, numerous experiments have been made to study the involvement of NF-κB in proliferation of this cell type. Numerous evidences suggest that in steps of atherosclerotic lesion formation, there are smooth muscle cell modifications, which changes from a contractile to a synthetic phenotype, these cells then displaying features similar to fibroblast and are the major source of connective tissue in this pathology [60, 61]. In cell cultures, smooth muscle cells in the synthetic state express genes that can be modulated by NF-κB, as tumor necrosis factor-α (TNF-α), interleukin 1 (IL-1), macrophage-colony stimulating factor (M-CSF), granulocyte macrophage-colony stimulating factor (GMCSF), or monocyte chemotactic protein–1 [60, 62–66].

The NF-κB involved in regulation of these genes may be activated by inflammatory cytokines or reactive oxygen intermediates, all of which can be produced by smooth muscle cells themselves as well as by monocyte/macrophages, endothelial cells, or lymphocytes [60, 62, 67–69]. Increased activation of NF-κB could even be triggered in an autocrine loop by NF-κB-induced TNF-α or IL-1 itself [62, 64]. Activated NF-κB has been identified in cultured smooth muscle cells using electrophoretic mobility shift assays. Additionally, two recent studies demonstrate NF-κB activation in cultured smooth muscle cells by fibronectin and thrombin [70, 71].

Because NF-κB has been considered a potential therapeutic target of vascular diseases, many studies were performed to examine the effects of NF-κB inhibition on neointima formation following vascular injury. For example, adenovirus-mediated transfer of IκB super-repressor inhibited the development of intimal hyperplasia after vascular injury in rats in vivo. Likewise, double-stranded decoy oligonucleotides that bind NF-κB and keep it localized in the cytoplasm decreased injury-induced neointima formation in rats and pigs, [72, 73] as well as in-stent restenosis in hypercholesterolemic rabbits [74]. Moreover, antisense oligonucleotides that decrease p65 synthesis reduced neointima formation following carotid injury in rats [75]. Most recently, the NF-κB essential modulator-binding domain peptide, which can block the activation of the IκB kinase complex and therefore inhibit NF-κB activation, was also able to reduce injury-induced neointima formation in rats and in apolipoprotein E-deficient mice [76]. Although results of these studies suggest that NF-κB inhibition is an effective therapeutic approach for vascular diseases, the target cell types had been unclear because of the global inhibition of NF-κB activity in these studies. In this regard, results of the study of Yoshida et al. (2005) [77] provide compelling evidence that NF-κB activation within smooth muscle cells is critical for injury-induced SMC phenotypic switching and neointima formation, although they do not negate a possibility that paracrine factors secreted by endothelial cells and/or monocytes/macrophages also affect the characteristics of smooth muscle cells. In fact, NF-κB inhibition in endothelial cells and macrophages has also been shown to decrease the formation of atherosclerosis [78]. Probably, NF-κB activation in multiple cell types including smooth muscle cells would simultaneously enhance lesion formation [79].

6. NF-κB in advanced lesions

In later stages of atherosclerosis, cell death became an important point. Death of lipid-laden cells is considered as an important step in the determination of the stability of the lesion and the formation of the necrotic core. Macrophage death by apoptosis, a prominent feature of atherosclerotic plaques, occurs in all stages of atherosclerosis and has a critical role in atherogenesis and atheroprogression [80]. Macrophage apoptosis in early lesions, coupled with rapid phagocytic clearance of dead cells (efferocytosis), reduces macrophage burden and slows lesion progression. Whereas in late lesions, macrophage apoptosis, accompanied by defective efferocytosis, promotes the enlargement of lipid core and results in inflammation, necrosis, and even plaque rupture, which are identified as the causative processes in the small percentage of atherosclerotic lesions that cause acute vascular events such as stroke, acute myocardial infarction, and sudden coronary death [81–84].

In atherosclerosis, NF-κB pathway regulates cell survival signaling by the inhibition of programmed cell death induced via TNF-receptors and several other triggers. The contribution of NF-κB to apoptosis is mediated through regulation of ROS production and a control of sustained activation of the c-Jun NH2-terminal kinases (JNK)-mitogen-activated protein kinases (MAPK) cascade [85, 86]. Generally, NF-κB pathway, by interfering with induction of ROS and JNK signaling, inhibits the apoptotic response and promotes cell survival, while its blockade induces oxidative stress and activation of JNK-MAPK cascade that results in cell death, via apoptosis or necrosis [87, 88].

The pro-survival activity of NF-κB is mediated by the phosphorylation and degradation of the inhibitory IκBα proteins through IκB kinase (IKK) [15, 87]. Ottonello et al. showed that a long-acting nonsteroidal anti-inflammatory drug, oxaprozin, is able to inhibit the activation of kinase Akt in human monocytes, mediated by immune complexes, and prevents the activation of NF-κB mediated by IKK. This inhibition leads to cell programmed cell death by the reduction of the production of the anti-apoptotic molecule X-linked mammalian inhibitor of apoptosis protein in monocytes [87, 89]. These antiapoptotic effects of NF-κB are sustained by a positive feedback regulation with TNFα, and are important in the pathogenesis of chronic inflammatory diseases (i.e., rheumatoid arthritis, inflammatory bowel disease) [14, 87, 90, 91]. Other evidences indicate that an aberrant NF-κB mediated inhibition of programmed cell death may be involved in the initiation of type-II diabetes and atherosclerosis [14, 87, 92, 93]. Anyhow, there are studies suggesting pro-apoptotic properties of NF-κB. It has been established that the activation of NF-κB increases expression of Fas ligand; the death factor Fas (CD95) is noted to contributing in cell apoptosis induced by DNA damage and other stresses. Thus, we can conclude that NF-κB is able to exert both pro- and anti-apoptotic properties depending upon the context of the various activating stimuli [87, 94].

Thrombosis associated with plaque rupture or erosion is the most acute complication of atherosclerosis and is an important mechanism in cardiovascular diseases, such as unstable angina and acute myocardial infarction. Several molecules have emerged as leading pathophysiological contributors, including thrombogenic tissue factor (TF), which is considered as the main initiator of coagulation and thrombus formation. In the last steps of atherosclerosis, the TF expression leads to activation of matrix metalloproteinase (MMP), which induces the loss of fibrous cap integrity, by collagen fibrils degradation, and infiltration and activation of inflammatory cells by pro-inflammatory cytokines. The expression of these mediators is regulated by transcription factors, such as NF-κB. TF, member of the cytokine receptor superfamily activates the coagulation cascade, forming a complex which cleaves factors IX and X, and thereby acts as an essential co-factor for factor VII/VIIa [3, 95, 96]. In human atherosclerotic vessels, different cells express TF, such as macrophages, smooth muscle cells, and endothelial cells that cover the plaque, but this factor is also present in the extracellular matrix. The TF promoter region presents a non-consensus NF-κB-binding site, which differs from the consensus sequence for one base [3, 97]. Lipopolysaccharide-mediated activation of TF transcription is inhibited by protease inhibitors of the chloromethylketone class in human monocytic cells, possibly preventing degradation of IκB [3, 98]. An inhibitor of the NF-κB pathway, the pyrrolidine dithiocarbamate, has the same effect on TF synthesis in endothelial cells modulated by different inducers [99]. TF is also inhibited in endothelial cells by the overexpression of IκBα or a dominant negative form of IKK-2 [100]. Recently, in fish, it has been demonstrated that in monocytes/macrophages the intracellular signaling pathways regulating TF is modulated by NF-κB [101].

Macrophages present in atherosclerotic plaques constitutively express MMP-1, -3, and -9, so the induction of these matrix-degrading enzymes is an important step inducing loss of fibrous cap integrity by the reduction of collagen protein [3, 102]. The release of MMP is regulated by NF-κB, but this may depend on the cell type and stimulus involved [103–105]. However, spontaneous secretion of MMP-9 by human macrophages does not appear to involve NF-κB, although Chase et al. demonstrated that NF-κB is a key factor in macrophage-derived MMP-1 and MMP-3 secretion. Inhibition of NF-κB dramatically reduced MMP-1 secretion from healthy human macrophages in response to CD40 ligation, a surface molecule in which ligation leads to this cells activation. Moreover, NF-κB was necessary for the pathology-related upregulation of MMP-1 and MMP-3 in foam cells elicited during atherosclerosis formation in vivo, thereby giving an indirect indication of the likely impact of NF-κB inhibition in vivo

[106]. Moreover, oxLDL, typical of atherosclerosis, has been found to increase macrophage MMP-9, associated with increased nuclear binding of NF-κB and activator protein-1 [13, 104].

7. Conclusions

Atherosclerosis and its complications are the major causes of mortality and morbidity around the world; for this reason, interventions aimed to prevent and treat these diseases are still a clinical challenge. Several researches suggest that the biology of the plaque is the first responsible for clinical manifestations of atherosclerosis. Current evidence supports a central role for inflammatory signaling pathways in all phases of the disease. Substantial biological data implicate NF-κB inflammatory pathways in early atherogenesis, in the progression of lesions, and finally in the thrombotic complications of this disease (Figure 1). This new insight into the role of NF-κB and of inflammation in the pathogenesis of atherosclerosis has initiated important new areas of direct clinical relevance. Future researches will be useful as guides to the development of inhibitors specific for the NF-κB pathway. Because the inhibitors now available lack of specificity for counteracting NF-κB activation eviting side effects, there is a need to identify appropriate therapeutic targets in the pathway for obtaining specific inhibition.

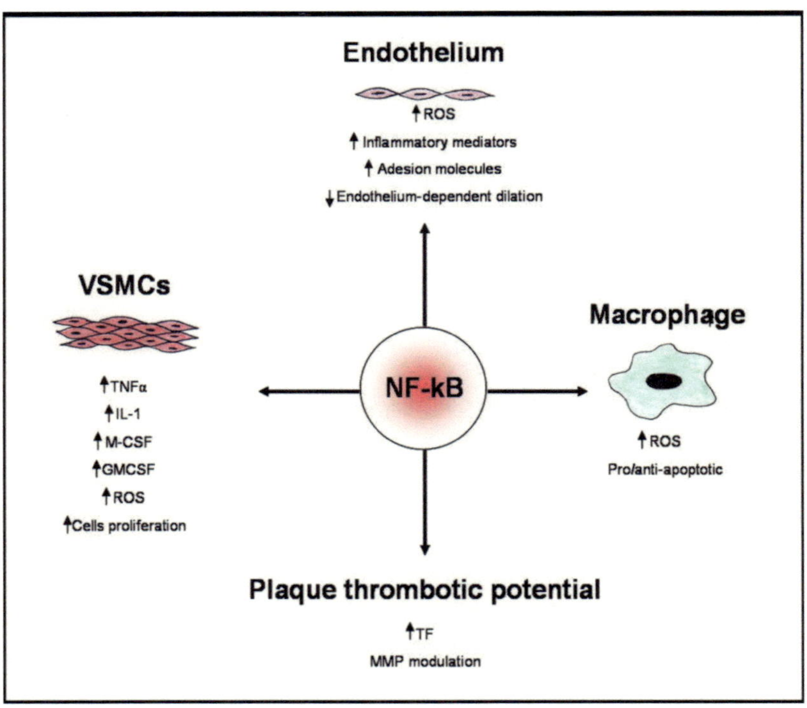

Figure 1. Representative image of the role of NF-κB in atherosclerosis

http://dx.doi.org/10.5772/61894

Nevertheless, the possibilities offered by a deeper understanding of the regulation of inflammatory signaling, including not just NF-κB but also other pathways, open up the promise of specific inhibition of disregulated inflammatory mechanisms causing disease.

Author details

Francesca Bonomini, Gaia Favero and Rita Rezzani*

*Address all correspondence to: rita.rezzani@unibs.it

Division of Anatomy and Physiopathology, Department of Clinical and Experimental Sciences, University of Brescia, Brescia, Italy

References

[1] Ross R. Atherosclerosis is an inflammatory disease. Am Heart J 1999;138:419–20.

[2] Husain K, Hernandez W, Ansari RA, Ferder L. Inflammation, oxidative stress and renin angiotensin system in atherosclerosis. World J Biol Chem 2015;6:209–17.

[3] Monaco C, Paleolog E. Nuclear factor kappaB: a potential therapeutic target in atherosclerosis and thrombosis. Cardiovasc Res 2004;61:671–82.

[4] Stary HC, Chandler AB, Glagov S, Guyton JR, Insull W Jr, Rosenfeld ME, Schaffer SA, Schwartz CJ, Wagner WD, Wissler RW. A definition of initial, fatty streak, and intermediate lesions of atherosclerosis. A report from the Committee on Vascular Lesions of the Council on Arteriosclerosis, American Heart Association. Circulation 1994;89:2462–78.

[5] Wöbke TK, Sorg BL, Steinhilber D. Vitamin D in inflammatory diseases. Front Physiol 2014;5:244.

[6] Toutouzas K, Synetos A, Nikolaou C, Tsiamis E, Tousoulis D, Stefanadis C. Matrix metalloproteinases and vulnerable atheromatous plaque. Curr Top Med Chem 2012;12:1166–80.

[7] Favero G, Rodella LF, Reiter RJ, Rezzani R. Melatonin and its atheroprotective effects: a review. Mol Cell Endocrinol 2014 Feb 15;382(2):926–37.

[8] Libby P, Lichtman AH, Hansson GK. Immune effector mechanisms implicated in atherosclerosis: from mice to humans. Immunity 2013;38:1092–104.

[9] Libby P. Mechanisms of acute coronary syndromes and their implication for therapy. N Engl J Med 2013;368:2004–13.

[10] Bentzon JF, Otsuka F, Virmani R, Falk E. Mechanisms of plaque formation and rupture. Circ Res 2014;114:1852–66.

[11] Yamashita T, Sasaki N, Kasahara K, Hirata KI. Anti-inflammatory and immune-modulatory therapies for preventing atherosclerotic cardiovascular disease. J Cardiol 2015;5087(15):36–42.

[12] Ghosh S, May MJ, Kopp EB. NF-kappa B and Rel proteins: evolutionarily conserved mediators of immune responses. Annu Rev Immunol 1998;16:225–60.

[13] Pahl HL. Activators and target genes of Rel/NF-kappaB transcription factors. Oncogene 1999;18:6853–66.

[14] Kumar A, Takada Y, Boriek AM, Aggarwal BB. Nuclear factor-kappaB: its role in health and disease. J Mol Med (Berl) 2004;82(7):434–48.

[15] Li Q, Verma IM. NF-kappaB regulation in the immune system. Nat Rev Immunol 2002;2:725–34.

[16] Senftleben U, Karin M. The IKK/NF-kappaB pathway. Crit Care Med 2002;30:18–26.

[17] Silverman N, Maniatis T. NF-kappaB signaling pathways in mammalian and insect innate immunity. Genes Dev 2001;15:2321–42.

[18] Karin M, Delhase M. The I kappa B kinase (IKK) and NF-kappa B: key elements of proinflammatory signaling. Semin Immunol 2000;12:85–98.

[19] Karin M, Lin A. NF-kappaB at the crossroads of life and death. Nat Immunol 2002;3:221–7.

[20] Kumar A, Lnu S, Malya R, Barron D, Moore J, Corry DB, Boriek AM. Mechanical stretch activates nuclear factor-kappaB, activator protein-1, and mitogen-activated protein kinases in lung parenchyma: implications in asthma. FASEB J 2003;17:1800–11.

[21] Kumar A, Boriek AM. Mechanical stress activates the nuclear factor-kappaB pathway in skeletal muscle fibers: a possible role in Duchenne muscular dystrophy. FASEB J 2003;17:386–96.

[22] Karin M, Ben-Neriah Y. Regulatory functions of ubiquitination in the immune system. Nat Immunol 2002;3:20–6.

[23] Wilkinson KD. Signal transduction: aspirin, ubiquitin and cancer. Nature 2003;424:738–9.

[24] Collins T, Cybulsky MI. NF-kappaB: pivotal mediator or innocent bystander in atherogenesis? J Clin Invest 2001;107:255–64.

[25] Brand K, Page S, Walli AK, Neumeier D, Baeuerle PA. Role of nuclear factor-kappa B in atherogenesis. Exp Physiol 1997;82:297–304.

[26] Boring L, Gosling J, Cleary M, Charo IF. Decreased lesion formation in CCR2-/- mice reveals a role for chemokines in the initiation of atherosclerosis. Nature 1998;394:894–7.

[27] Cybulsky MI, Gimbrone MAJ. Endothelial expression of a mononuclear leukocyte adhesion molecule during atherogenesis. Science 1991;251:788–91.

[28] Iiyama K, Hajra L, Iiyama M, Li H, DiChiara M, Medoff BD, Cybulsky MI. Patterns of vascular cell adhesion molecule-1 and intercellular adhesion molecule-1 expression in rabbit and mouse atherosclerotic lesions and at sites predisposed to lesion formation. Circ Res 1999;85:199–207.

[29] Brand K, Page S, Rogler G, Bartsch A, Brandl R, Knuechel R, Page M, Kaltschmidt C, Baeuerle PA, Neumeier D. Activated transcription factor nuclear factor-kappa B is present in the atherosclerotic lesion. J Clin Invest 1996;97:1715–22.

[30] Wilson SH, Caplice NM, Simari RD, Holmes DRJ, Carlson PJ, Lerman A. Activated nuclear factor-kappaB is present in the coronary vasculature in experimental hypercholesterolemia. Atherosclerosis 2000;148:23–30.

[31] Hernandez-Presa MA, Ortego M, Tunon J, Martin-Ventura JL, Mas S, Blanco-Colio LM, Aparicio C, Ortega L, Gomez-Gerique J, Vivanco F, Egido J. Simvastatin reduces NF-kappaB activity in peripheral mononuclear and in plaque cells of rabbit atheroma more markedly than lipid lowering diet. Cardiovasc Res 2003;57:168–77.

[32] Gradinaru D, Borsa C, Ionescu C, Prada GI. Oxidized LDL and NO synthesis: biomarkers of endothelial dysfunction and ageing. Mech Ageing Dev 2015;6374(15):28–37.

[33] Simionescu M, Antohe F. Functional ultrastructure of the vascular endothelium: changes in various pathologies. Handb Exp Pharmacol 2006;176:41–69.

[34] Mehta D, Malik AB. Signaling mechanisms regulating endothelial permeability. Physiol Rev 2006;86(1):279–367.

[35] Sima AV, Stancu CS, Simionescu M. Vascular endothelium in atherosclerosis. Cell Tissue Res 2009;335(1):191–203.

[36] Donato AJ, Morgan RG, Walker AE, Lesniewski LA. Cellular and molecular biology of aging endothelial cells. J Mol Cell Cardiol 2015;2828(15):34–6.

[37] Lesniewski LA, Durrant JR, Connell ML, Folian BJ, Donato AJ, Seals DR. Salicylate treatment improves age-associated vascular endothelial dysfunction: potential role of nuclear factor kappaB and forkhead Box O phosphorylation. J Gerontol A Biol Sci Med Sci 2011;66(4):409–18.

[38] Walker AE, Kaplon RE, Pierce GL, Nowlan MJ, Seals DR. Prevention of age-related endothelial dysfunction by habitual aerobic exercise in healthy humans: possible role of nuclear factor κB. Clin Sci (Lond) 2014;127(11):645–54.

[39] Pierce GL, Lesniewski LA, Lawson BR, Beske SD, Seals DR. Nuclear factor-{kappa}B activation contributes to vascular endothelial dysfunction via oxidative stress in overweight/obese middle-aged and older humans. Circulation 2009;119(9):1284–92.

[40] Csiszar A, Smith K, Labinskyy N, Orosz Z, Rivera A, Ungvari Z. Resveratrol attenuates TNF-alpha-induced activation of coronary arterial endothelial cells: role of NF-kappaB inhibition. Am J Physiol Heart Circ Physiol 2006;291(4):1694–9.

[41] Xiao J, Song J, Hodara V, Ford A, Wang XL, Shi Q, Chen L, Vandeberg JL. Protective effects of Resveratrol on TNF-α-induced endothelial cytotoxicity in baboon femoral Arterial endothelial cells. J Diabetes Res 2013;2013:185172–80.

[42] Donato AJ, Henson GD, Morgan RG, Enz RA, Walker AE, Lesniewski LA. TNF-α impairs endothelial function in adipose tissue resistance arteries of mice with diet-induced obesity. Am J Physiol Heart Circ Physiol 2012;303(6):672–9.

[43] Gareus R, Kotsaki E, Xanthoulea S, Van der Made I, Gijbels MJ, Kardakaris R, Polykratis A, Kollias G, de Winther MP, Pasparakis M. Endothelial cell-specific NF-kappaB inhibition protects mice from atherosclerosis. Cell Metab 2008;8(5):372–83.

[44] Bjorkbacka H, Kunjathoor VV, Moore KJ, Koehn S, Ordija CM, Lee MA, Means T, Halmen K, Luster AD, Golenbock DT, Freeman MW. Reduced atherosclerosis in MyD88-null mice links elevated serum cholesterol levels to activation of innate immunity signaling pathways. Nat Med 2004;10:416–21.

[45] Mullick AE, Soldau K, Kiosses WB, Bell TA, III Tobias PS, Curtiss LK. Increased endothelial expression of Toll-like receptor 2 at sites of disturbed blood flow exacerbates early atherogenic events. J Exp Med 2008;205:373–83.

[46] Miller YI, Viriyakosol S, Binder CJ, Feramisco JR, Kirkland TN, Witztum JL. Minimally modified LDL binds to CD14, induces macrophage spreading via TLR4/MD-2, and inhibits phagocytosis of apoptotic cells. J Biol Chem 2003;278:1561–8.

[47] Miller YI, Viriyakosol S, Worrall DS, Boullier A, Butler S, Witztum JL. Toll-like receptor 4-dependent and -independent cytokine secretion induced by minimally oxidized low-density lipoprotein in macrophages. Arterioscler Thromb Vasc Biol 20055;25:1213–9.

[48] Michelsen KS, Wong MH, Shah PK, Zhang W, Yano J, Doherty TM, Akira S, Rajavashisth TB, Arditi M. Lack of Toll-like receptor 4 or myeloid differentiation factor 88 reduces atherosclerosis and alters plaque phenotype in mice deficient in apolipoprotein E. Proc Natl Acad Sci USA 2004;101:10679–84.

[49] Hajra L, Evans AI, Chen M, Hyduk SJ, Collins T, Cybulsky MI. The NF-kappa B signal transduction pathway in aortic endothelial cells is primed for activation in regions predisposed to atherosclerotic lesion formation. Proc Natl Acad Sci USA 2000;97:9052–7.

[50] Orr AW, Sanders JM, Bevard M, Coleman E, Sarembock IJ, Schwartz MA. The subendothelial extracellular matrix modulates NF-kappaB activation by flow: a potential role in atherosclerosis. J Cell Biol 2005;169:191–202.

[51] Manea A, Manea SA, Gafencu AV, Raicu M. Regulation of NADPH oxidase subunit p22(phox) by NF-κB in human aortic smooth muscle cells. Arch Physiol Biochem 2007;113:163–72.

[52] Kuwano Y, Kawahara T, Yamamoto H, Teshima-Kondo S, Tominaga K, Masuda K, et al. Interferon-gamma activates transcription of NADPH oxidase 1 gene and upregulates production of superoxide anion by human large intestinal epithelial cells. Am J Physiol Cell Physiol 2006;290:433–43.

[53] Anrather J, Racchumi G, Iadecola C. NF-kappaB regulates phagocytic NADPH oxidase by inducing the expression of gp91phox. J Biol Chem 2006;281:5657–67.

[54] Osterud B, Bjorklid E. Role of monocytes in atherogenesis. Physiol Rev 2003;83(4): 1069–112.

[55] Brand K, Eisele T, Kreusel U, Page M, Page S, Haas M, Gerling A, Kaltschmidt C, Neumann FJ, Mackman N, Baeurele PA, Walli AK, Neumeier D. Dysregulation of monocytic nuclear factor-kappa B by oxidized low-density lipoprotein. Arterioscler Thromb Vasc Biol 1997;17:1901–9.

[56] Khan BV, Parthasarathy SS, Alexander RW, Medford RM. Modified low-density lipoprotein and its constituents augment cytokineactivated vascular cell adhesion molecule-1 gene expression in human vascular endothelial cells. J Clin Invest 1995;95:1262–70.

[57] Palmetshofer A, Robson SC, Nehls V. Lysophosphatidic acid activates nuclear factor kappa B and induces proinflammatory gene expression in endothelial cells. Thromb Haemost 1999;82:1532–7.

[58] Calara F, Dimayuga P, Niemann A, Thyberg J, Diczfalusy U, Witztum JL, Palinski W, Shah PK, Cercek B, Nilsson J, Regnström J. An animal model to study local oxidation of LDL and its biological effects in the arterial wall. Arterioscler Thromb Vasc Biol 1998;18:884–93.

[59] Dichtl W, Nilsson L, Goncalves I, Ares MP, Banfi C, Calara F, Hamsten A, Eriksson P, Nilsson J. Very low-density lipoprotein activates nuclear factor-kappaB in endothelial cells. Circ Res 1999;84:1085–94.

[60] Ross R. The pathogenesis of atherosclerosis: a perspective for the 1990s. Nature (Lond) 1993;362:801–9.

[61] Amento EP, Ehsani N, Palmer H, Libby P. Cytokines and growth factors positively and negatively regulate interstitial collagen gene expression in human vascular smooth muscle cells. Arterioscler Thromb 1991;11:1223–30.

[62] Baeuerle PA, Henkel T. Function and activation of NF-κB in the immune system. Annu Rev Immunol 1994;12:141–79.

[63] Barath P, Fishbein MC, Lao J, Bernson J, Helfaut RH, Forrester JS. Tumor necrosis factor gene expression in human vascular smooth muscle cells detected by in vitro hybridization. Am J Pathol 1990;137:503–9.

[64] Hiscott J, Marois J, Garoufalis J, D'Addarion M, Roulston A, Kwan I, Pepin N, Lacoste J, Nguyen H, Bensi G, Fenton M. Characterization of a functional NF-kappa B site in the human interleukin-1b promoter: evidence for a positive autoregulatory loop. Mol Cell Biol 1993;13:6231–40.

[65] Rosenfeld ME, Ylä-Herttuala S, Lipton BA, Ord VA, Witztum JL, Steinberg D. Macrophage colony-stimulating factor mRNA and protein in atherosclerotic lesions of rabbits and humans. Am J Pathol 1992;140:291–300.

[66] Clinton SK, Underwood R, Haynes L, Sherman ML, Kufe DW, Libby P. Macrophage colony-stimulating factor gene expression in vascular cells and in experimental and human atherosclerosis. Am J Pathol 1992;140:301–16.

[67] Müller JM, Ziegler-Heitbrock HWL, Baeuerle PA. Nuclear factor kappa B, a mediator of lipopolysaccharide effects. Immunobiology 1993;187:233–56.

[68] Witztum JL, Steinberg D. Role of oxidized low density lipoprotein in atherogenesis. J Clin Invest 1991;88:1785–92.

[69] Berliner JA, Territo M, Andalibi A, Navab M, Liao F, Cushing S, Imes S, Kim J, Van Lenten B, Lusis AJ, Fogelman AM. Modified lipoproteins and atherogenesis. In: Gotto JAM. (Ed.) Cellular and Molecular Biology of Atherosclerosis. Springer-Verlag London Ltd., London. 1992. Pp. 77–80.

[70] Qwarnström EE, Ostberg CO, Turk GL, Richardson CA, Bomsztyk K. Fibronectin attachment activates the NF-κB p50/p65 heterodimer in fibroblasts and smooth muscle cells. J Biol Chem 1994;269:30765–8.

[71] Nakajima T, Kitajima I, Shin H, Takasaki I, Shigeta K, Abeyama K, Yamashita Y, Tokioka T, Soejima Y, Maruyama I. Involvement of NF-κB activation in thrombin-induced human vascular smooth muscle cell proliferation. Biochem Biophys Res Commun 1994;204:950–5.

[72] Yoshimura S, Morishita R, Hayashi K, Yamamoto K, Nakagami H, Kaneda Y, Sakai N, Ogihara T. Inhibition of intimal hyperplasia after balloon injury in rat carotid artery model using cis-element "decoy" of nuclear factor-κB binding site as a novel molecular strategy. Gene Ther 2001;8:1635–42.

[73] Yamasaki K, Asai T, Shimizu M, Aoki M, Hashiya N, Sakonjo H, Makino H, Kaneda Y, Ogihara T, Morishita R. Inhibition of NFjB activation using ciselement "decoy" of NFjB binding site reduces neointimal formation in porcine balloon-injured coronary artery model. Gene Ther 2003;10:356–64.

[74] Ohtani K, Egashira K, Nakano K, Zhao G, Funakoshi K, Ihara Y, Kimura S, Tominaga R, Morishita R, Sunagawa K. Stent-based local delivery of nuclear factor-jB decoy attenuates in-stent restenosis in hypercholesterolemic rabbits. Circulation 2006;114:2773–9.

[75] Autieri MV, Yue TL, Ferstein GZ, Ohlstein E. Antisense oligonucleotides to the p65 subunit of NF-jB inhibit human vascular smooth muscle cell adherence and proliferation and prevent neointima formation in rat carotid arteries. Biochem Biophys Res Commun 1995;213:827–36.

[76] Grassia G, Maddaluno M, Musilli C, De Stefano D, Carnuccio R, Di Lauro MV, Parratt CA, Kennedy S, Di Meglio P, Ianaro A, Maffia P, Parenti A, Ialenti A. The IjB kinase inhibitor nuclear factor-jB essential modulator-binding domain peptide for inhibition of injury-induced neointimal formation. Arterioscler Thromb Vasc Biol 2010;30:2458–66.

[77] Yoshida T, Owens GK. Molecular determinants of vascular smooth muscle cell diversity. Circ Res 2005;96(3):280–91.

[78] Kanters E, Gijbels MJ, van der Made I, Vergouwe MN, Heeringa P, Kraal G, Hofker MH, de Winther MP. Hematopoietic NF-jB1 deficiency results in small atherosclerotic lesions with an inflammatory phenotype. Blood 2004;103:934–40.

[79] Yoshida T, Yamashita M, Horimai C, Hayashi M. Smooth muscle-selective inhibition of nuclear factor-κB attenuates smooth muscle phenotypic switching and neointima formation following vascular injury. J Am Heart Assoc 2013;2(3):230–3.

[80] Moore KJ, Tabas I. Macrophages in the pathogenesis of atherosclerosis. Cell 2011;29;145(3):341–55.

[81] Tabas I. Consequences and therapeutic implications of macrophage apoptosis in atherosclerosis: the importance of lesion stage and phagocytic efficiency. Arterioscler Thromb Vasc Biol 2005;25(11):2255–64.

[82] Tabas I. Macrophage death and defective inflammation resolution in atherosclerosis. Nat Rev Immunol 2010;10(1):36–46.

[83] Littlewood TD, Bennett MR. Apoptotic cell death in atherosclerosis. Curr Opin Lipidol 2003;14(5):469–75.

[84] Yao S, Tian H, Miao C, Zhang DW, Zhao L, Li Y, Yang N, Jiao P, Sang H, Guo S, Wang Y, Qin S. D4F alleviates macrophage-derived foam cell apoptosis by inhibiting endoplasmic reticulum stress-CHOP pathway. J Lipid Res 2015 [Epub ahead of print].

[85] Bubici C, Papa S, Pham CG, Zazzeroni F, Franzoso G. NF-kappaB and JNK: an intricate affair. Cell Cycle 2004;3(12):1524–9.

[86] Luo JL, Kamata H, Karin M. IKK/NF-kappaB signaling: balancing life and death-a new approach to cancer therapy. J Clin Invest 2005;115(10):2625–32.

[87] Pamukcu B, Lip GY, Shantsila E. The nuclear factor--kappa B pathway in atherosclerosis: a potential therapeutic target for atherothrombotic vascular disease. Thromb Res 2011;128(2):117–23.

[88] Papa S, Bubici C, Zazzeroni F, Pham CG, Kuntzen C, Knabb JR, Dean K, Franzoso G. The NF-kappaB-mediated control of the JNK cascade in the antagonism of programmed cell death in health and disease. Cell Death Differ 2006;13(5):712–29.

[89] Ottonello L, Bertolotto M, Montecucco F, Bianchi G, Dallegri F. Delayed apoptosis of human monocytes exposed to immune complexes is reversed by oxaprozin: role of the Akt/IkappaB kinase/nuclear factor kappaB pathway. Br J Pharmacol 2009;157(2): 294–306.

[90] Kucharczak J, Simmons MJ, Fan Y., Gelinas C. To be, or not to be: NF-κB is the answer – role of Rel/NF-κB in the regulation of apoptosis. Oncogene 2003;56:8961–82.

[91] Liu H, Pope R.M. The role of apoptosis in rheumatoid arthritis. Curr Opin Pharmacol 2003;3:317–22.

[92] Shoelson SE, Lee J, Yuan M. Inflammation and the IKκB/IκB/NFκB axis in obesity- and diet-induced insulin resistance. Int J Obes Relat Metab Disord 2003;3:S49–52.

[93] Dandona P, Aljada A, Chaudhuri A, Mohanty P, Garg R. Metabolic syndrome: a comprehensive perspective based on interactions between obesity, diabetes, and inflammation. Circulation 2005;111:1448–54.

[94] Kasibhatla S, Brunner T, Genestier L, Echeverri F, Mahboubi A, Green DR. DNA damaging agents induce expression of Fas ligand and subsequent apoptosis in T lymphocytes via the activation of NF-κB and AP-1. Mol Cell 1998;1:543–51.

[95] Nemerson Y. Tissue factor: then and now. Thromb Haemost 1995;74(1):180–4.

[96] Zoldhelyi P, Chen ZQ, Shelat HS, McNatt JM, Willerson JT. Local gene transfer of tissue factor pathway inhibitor regulates intimal hyperplasia in atherosclerotic arteries. Proc Natl Acad Sci USA 2001; 98:4078–83.

[97] Mackman N, Morrissey JH, Fowler B, Edgington TS. Complete sequence of the human tissue factor gene, a highly regulated cellular receptor that initiates the coagulation protease cascade. Biochemistry 1989;28:1755–62.

[98] Mackman N. Protease inhibitors block lipopolysaccharide induction of tissue factor gene expression in human monocytic cells by preventing activation of c-Rel/p65 heterodimers. J Biol Chem 1994;269:26363–7.

[99] Orthner CL, Rodgers GM, Fitzgerald LA. Pyrrolidine dithiocarbamate abrogates tissue factor (TF) expression by endothelial cells: evidence implicating nuclear factor-kappa B in TF induction by diverse agonists. Blood 1995;86:436–43.

[100] Wrighton CJ, Hofer-Warbinek R, Moll T, Eytner R, Bach FH, de Martin R. Inhibition of endothelial cell activation by adenovirus-mediated expression of I- kappa B alpha, an inhibitor of the transcription factor NF-kappa B. J Exp Med 1996;183:1013–22.

[101] Wei H, Yin L, Feng S, Wang X, Yang K, Zhang A, Zhou H. Dual-parallel inhibition of IL-10 and TGF-β1 controls LPS-induced inflammatory response via NF-κB signaling in grass carp monocytes/macrophages. Fish Shellfish Immunol 2015;44(2):445–52.

[102] Galis ZS, Sukhova GK, Lark MW, Libby P. Increased expression of matrix metalloproteinases and matrix degrading activity in vulnerable regions of human atherosclerotic plaques. J Clin Invest 1994;94:2493–503.

[103] Bond M, Fabunmi RP, Baker AH, Newby AC. Synergistic upregulation of metalloproteinase-9 by growth factors and inflammatory cytokines: an absolute requirement for transcription factor NF-kappa B. FEBS Lett 1998;435:29–34.

[104] Bond M., Chase AJ, Baker AH, Newby AC. Inhibition of transcription factor NF-kappaB reduces matrix metalloproteinase-1, -3 and -9 production by vascular smooth muscle cells. Cardiovasc Res 2001;50:556–65.

[105] Feldmann M, Andreakos E, Smith C, Bondeson J, Yoshimura S, Kiriakidis S, Monaco C, Gasparini C, Sacre S, Lundberg A, Paleolog E, Horwood NJ, Brennan FM, Foxwell BM. Is NF-kappaB a useful therapeutic target in rheumatoid arthritis? Ann Rheum Dis 2002;61(Suppl 2):ii13–8.

[106] Chase AJ, Bond M, Crook MF, Newby AC. Role of nuclear factor-kappa B activation in metalloproteinase-1, -3, and -9 secretion by human macrophages in vitro and rabbit foam cells produced in vivo. Arterioscler Thromb Vasc Biol 2002;22(5):765–71.

[107] Xu XP, Meisel SR, Ong JM, Kaul S, Cercek B, Rajavashisth TB, Sharifi B, Shah PK. Oxidized low-density lipoprotein regulates matrix metalloproteinase-9 and its tissue inhibitor in human monocyte-derived macrophages. Circulation 1999;99(8):993–8.

Chapter 3

Thrombosis, Atherosclerosis and Atherothrombosis – New Insights and Experimental Protocols

Jasmina Dimitrova-Shumkovska, Leo Veenman, Inbar Roim, Svetlana Leschiner and Moshe Gavish

Additional information is available at the end of the chapter

http://dx.doi.org/10.5772/61971

Abstract

Previous studies have shown that TSPO as well as apolipoprotein E (Apo E) can be associated with processes such as cholesterol metabolism, oxidative stress, apoptosis, glial activation, inflammation, and immune responses. As a ligand for cell-surface lipoprotein receptors, apolipoprotein E can prevent atherosclerosis by clearing cholesterol-rich lipoproteins from plasma. Furthermore, TSPO takes part in the regulation of gene expression for proteins involved in adhesion, which potentially may play a role in platelet aggregation. There are indications that the Apo E protein is involve in platelet aggregation, while TSPO platelet levels have been found to be increased with various neurological disorders, in particular, in stress-related disorders. The role of platelets in atherogenesis and the potential therapeutic impact of TSPO ligands on disease prevention are of great interest. To determine TSPO binding characteristics in this paradigm, we applied binding assays with [^{3}H]PK 11195 on isolated platelets and erythrocyte membranes. The in vivo findings in Apo E knockout mice revealed that TSPO levels appear to be enhanced in platelets and erythrocytes of Apo E knockout mice, and thus suggest that TSPO and Apo E expression may be interconnected in relation to some aspect of the host defense response. Other organs tested, such as liver, testis, brain, heart, aorta, lung, kidney and spleen, did not show a difference in TSPO binding levels between Apo E knockout mice and wild-type mice. This suggests that TSPO levels may be part of a feedback control system for steroid production (responding to alterations in steroid levels), rather than being regulated by a feed-forward signal provided by cholesterol (i.e. TSPO levels in relation to steroidogenesis are not being regulated by cholesterol levels in vivo).

Keywords: Dyslipidemia, Platelets, Translocator protein, Erythrocytes, Apo E-KO mice

INTECH
open science | open minds

1. Introduction

1.1. The connection of apolipopoprotein E and platelet activation to inflammation and atherosclerosis

Atherosclerosis is a chronic inflammatory disease of the arteries of multifactorial etiology that involves a complex interaction among oxidized lipids, plasma proteins, vascular endothelial and smooth muscle cells and platelets [1–3]. Hypercholesterolemia and especially high concentrations of low-density lipoproteins (LDL) are significant factors for the premature development of atherosclerotic plaque. In parallel, elevated LDL levels exert prothrombotic effects via platelet activation [4].

Dysfunction or low levels of platelets predispose to bleeding, while high levels, although usually asymptomatic, may increase the risk of thrombosis, thus relating to atherosclerosis and Apo E malfunction [5]. Studies from Kolodgie et al. demonstrated that platelets and erythrocytes can penetrate the plaque through angiogenic capillary breakages [6]. Furthermore, platelets with their pro-atherogenic potential are regarded as discrete immune cells [7, 8]. They can accumulate lipids in the hypercholesterolemic environment and are involved in the early phase of atheromatous formation [9]. Oxidized low-density lipoproteins (ox-LDLs) are suggested to be implicated in the early phase of atherosclerosis by recruiting inflammatory cells in the subendothelium that elucidate the thrombotic process [10]. Several cells including endothelial cells, macrophages and smooth muscle cells determine ox-LDL formation. *In vitro* studies have shown that ox-LDL binds to platelets via CD36 and lectin-like endothelial receptor for ox-LDL (LOX-1 receptors), promoting platelet activation [11, 12]. Experimental studies demonstrated a marked reduction of thrombus formation in animals with the deletion of ox-LDL receptor CD36 from platelets [13]. In accordance with a number of *in vitro* results, *in vivo* LOX-1 expression, was not only upregulated under the influence of proinflammatory stimulus but also induced in adipose tissue after high-fat diet feeding, suggesting that increased LOX-1 expression may promote atherosclerosis [14, 15].

Apolipoprotein E functions as an important carrier protein in the redistribution of lipids among cells, by incorporating into high-density lipoproteins (as HDL-E), and plays a prominent role in the transport (by incorporating into intestinally synthesized chylomicrons) and metabolism of plasma cholesterol and triglyceride through its ability to interact with the LDLR and the receptor binding of Apo E lipoproteins (apoER) [16, 17]. The metabolic activity of Apo E is sensitive to its lipid environment; purified Apo E does not interact with the LDLR [18]. Apo E at the surfaces of VLDL and chylomicrons is also inactive unless these lipoproteins are from hypertriglyceridemic subjects [19] or have undergone substantial lipolysis to form remnant particles [20]. Apo E is part of different metabolic pathways in the body. One of these pathways is endocrine-like, and involves the redistribution of lipids among cells of different organs. It takes lipids from the areas where the lipid is synthesized and distributes them to other areas where the lipids are used or stored. Another pathway is paracrine-like, where the lipids are transported among cells in the same organ or tissue. Since Apo E is involved directly in the uptake and distribution of plasma lipids, it is natural that it has several implications for

http://dx.doi.org/10.5772/61971

cardiovascular disease. Interestingly, oxLDL as a ligand for LOX-1 is highly present in circulation and lesion formation in atherosclerotic prone animals, such as Apo E KO mice.

The Apo E is also involved in various pathways that are unrelated to lipid transport, such as the stimulation of lymphocytes and macrophage secretion [21]. This appears important for facilitating local cholesterol redistribution and for reverse cholesterol transport [22]. As a ligand for cell surface lipoprotein receptors, apolipoprotein E can prevent atherosclerosis by clearing cholesterol-rich lipoproteins from plasma. Indeed, atherosclerosis in Apo E-deficient (Apo E2/2) mice can be prevented by transplantation of normal murine bone marrow cells [23], by macrophage-specific expression of the human Apo E transgene [24], or by adenovirus-mediated gene replacement [25]. It was also found that altered Apo E expression leads to enhanced inflammation responses [26–28].

Defects in Apo E sometimes result in its inability to bind to the LDL receptors, which leads to an increase in a person's blood cholesterol. Recently, it has been suggested that high cholesterol levels due to Apo E malfunction may constitute a risk factor for Alzheimer's disease [29, 30]. According to the expressed isoforms, Apo E might be involved (i) in maintaining the integrity of the aging CNS [31]; (ii) in repair, growth and maintenance of myelin and axonal membranes during development and after an injury [32]; (iii) in neurite outgrowth [33]; (iv) in neurotoxicity [34]; and (v) in pathological processes in general, including Alzheimer's disease [35].

Riddell's study found that HDL-E was a powerful inhibitor of agonist-induced platelet aggregation, through interaction with saturable binding sites in the platelet surface membrane, which further suggested that Apo E exerts its antiplatelet aggregation effect via L-arginine: nitric oxide pathway by enhancing the production of endogenous nitric oxide (NO) [36]. Calcium is central to the control of platelet reactivity, interacting with diverse second messengers through a myriad of complex but tightly regulated, signalling pathways [37]. Two important control elements for suppression of platelet activation are the cyclic nucleotides, cyclic adenosine monophosphate (cAMP) and cyclic guanosine monophosphate (cGMP), and agents that increase their intraplatelet levels exert antiaggregatory effects both *in vitro* and *in vivo* [38]. Although Apo E induced increases in both cAMP and cGMP, additional experiments implicated a specific stimulation of guanylate cyclase activity and a rise in cGMP as prerequisites for the antiplatelet action of Apo E. Using the L-arginine:nitric oxide pathway, the vascular endothelium synthesizes NO from the terminal guanidine nitrogen atoms of L-arginine using a soluble enzyme called NO synthase (NOS). NO then binds to soluble guanylate cyclase to produce cGMP, which has inhibitory effects on platelet aggregation. The increased levels of cGMP also decrease the amount of cAMP phosphodiesterase, the enzyme that converts cAMP to AMP. The decrease in cAMP phosphodiesterase causes an increase in cAMP, and cAMP also has an inhibitory effect on platelet aggregation [10, 36].

1.2. Potential functional commonalities between apolipoprotein E and 18 kDa translocator protein

It was shown previously that the 18 kDa translocator protein (TSPO) is present throughout the cardiovascular system and may be involved in cardiovascular disorders such as ischemia [36]. At cellular levels, TSPO is present in virtually all of the cells of the cardiovascular system, where they appear to take part in the responses to various challenges that an organism and its cardiovascular system face, including atherosclerosis and accompanying symptoms [22, 39–42].

The TSPO was previously known as peripheral type benzodiazepine receptor (PBR), since it is capable of binding benzodiazepines and is found in most if not all peripheral tissues [43]. Mitochondrial membranes form the primary location for TSPO [44]. It is an integral membrane protein that interacts with a wide variety of endogenous ligands, such as cholesterol and porphyrins, and is also a target for several small molecules with substantial *in vivo* efficacy. When complexed with the TSPO-specific radioligand PK11195, TSPO folds into a rigid five-helix bundle.

TSPO are present in platelets, lymphocytes and mononuclear cells and are also found in the endothelium, the striated cardiac muscle, the vascular smooth muscles and the mast cells of the cardiovascular system. As TSPO is known to regulate heme metabolism, TSPO may play essential roles in erythrocyte function [45]. TSPO in the cardiovascular system also appears to play roles in several aspects of the immune response, such as phagocytosis and the secretion of interleukin-2, interleukin-3 and immunoglobulin A [46]. Mast cells are considered to be important for immune response to pathogens [47], and they have also been implicated in the regulation of thrombosis and inflammation and cardiovascular disease processes such as atherosclerosis as well as in neoplastic conditions [48]. Benzodiazepines have been found to bind to specific receptors on macrophages and to modulate *in vitro* their metabolic oxidative responsiveness [49]. Haemin, isolated from human erythrocytes, competitively inhibits mitochondrial benzodiazepine binding with a Ki of 41 nM [50]. The TSPO might present a therapeutic target for arrhythmia, myocardial infarction and cardiac hypertrophy by reducing ROS. For example, the suppression of TSPO can prevent caspase cascade activation and cytochrome *c* release, thus inhibiting ROS overload [5, 51–60]. The results from several *in vitro* studies have implicated TSPO in cholesterol transport into mitochondria, the late-limiting step in the steroid biosynthesis. Therefore, TSPO has been considered as a critical factor in steroidogenesis. Moreover, the ubiquitous expression and evolutionary conservation of TSPO from bacteria to mammals strongly suggested its essential role in cellular processes. This presumption was further supported by the results of an earlier study that claimed the embryonic lethality of TSPO whole-body knockout (KO) mice, although the details of the methods for the design and generation of the KO mice were not provided [52, 53].

A scheme of the involvement of mitochondrial TSPO in various cellular functions and disease is given in Figure 1. For detailed discussions regarding these functional pathways, see refs. [49] and [58].

TSPO molecules are often found in groups and in conjugation with VDAC and ANT. As indicated in the figure, pk10, PRAX-1 and PAP7 face the cytosol. Furthermore, molecules of the Bcl-2 family and creatine kinase and hexokinase can be attached to VDAC and ANT. Various synthetic ligands that bind to TSPO have been developed. Endogenous ligands that bind to TSPO include: protoporphyrin IX, DBI and its fragment TTN and PLA2. The TSPO is involved in various functions as indicated towards the bottom of the figure. Abbreviations: ANT, adenine nucleotide transporter; ATP, adenosine triphosphate; DBI, diazepam-binding

http://dx.doi.org/10.5772/61971

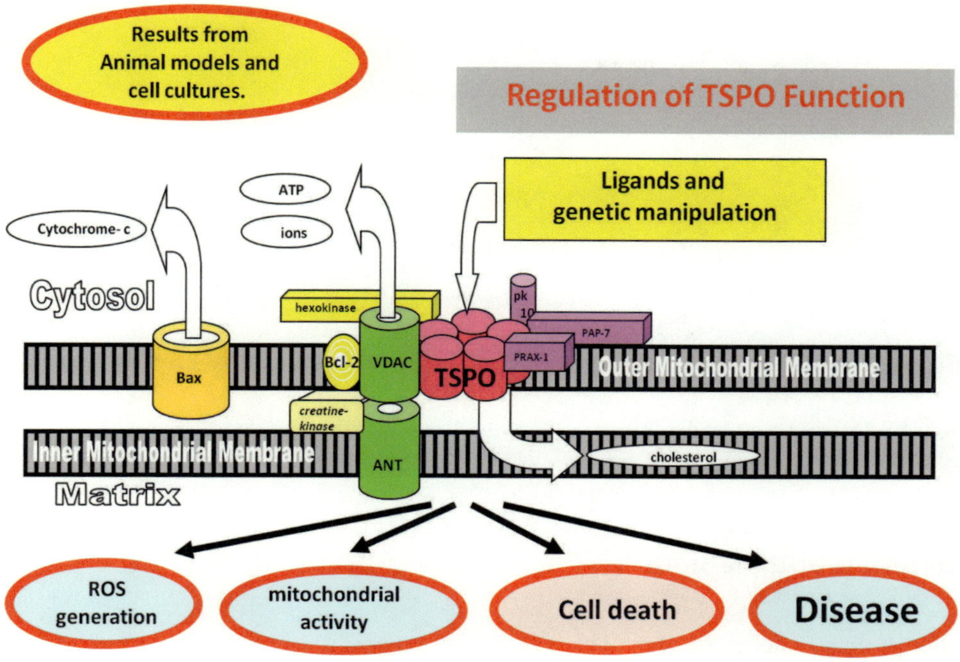

Figure 1. The 18 kDa mitochondrial translocator protein (TSPO) in relation to cellular function and disease.

inhibitor; PAP7, PBR-associated protein 7; PBR, peripheral-type benzodiazepine receptor; pk10, protein of 10 kilodalton; PLA2, phospholipase A2; PRAX-1, PBR-associated protein 1; TSPO, translocator protein (18 kDa); TTN, triakontatetraneuropeptide; VDAC, voltage-dependent anion channel.

Recently, it was shown that TSPO ligands specifically designed for this purpose can increase lifespan in animal models for human disease [61]. For example, the occurrence of cardiac arrest, the typical cause of death in R6-2 mice, is delayed considerably in this animal model for Huntington disease [62]. In numbers, average lifespan is increased from ±12 weeks to ±15 weeks. Translated to the human situation, this would mean in simple terms that life expectancy of Huntington disease patients can potentially be increased from an average of 60 years to an average of 85 years following treatments with the appropriate TSPO ligands. Such TSPO ligands were also shown to prevent and counteract brain edema associated with seizures developed after systemic injections of kainic acid in rats [61, 62].

Anti-inflammatory properties of TSPO ligands have also been demonstrated in nonneuronal tissues [63]. TSPO ligands have been shown to reduce inflammation in animal models of rheumatoid arthritis [59], carrageenan-induced pleurisy [64] and pulmonary inflammation [65]. A summary of the involvement of TSPO and apoE in functions common to both as suggested by previous studies discussed above is presented in Figure 2. Therefore, we studied whether knockout of apolipoprotein E in mice may have an effect on TSPO expression in platelets and erythrocytes. This could suggest that TSPO is involved in the regulation of functions under the control of ApoE as mentioned in Figure 2.

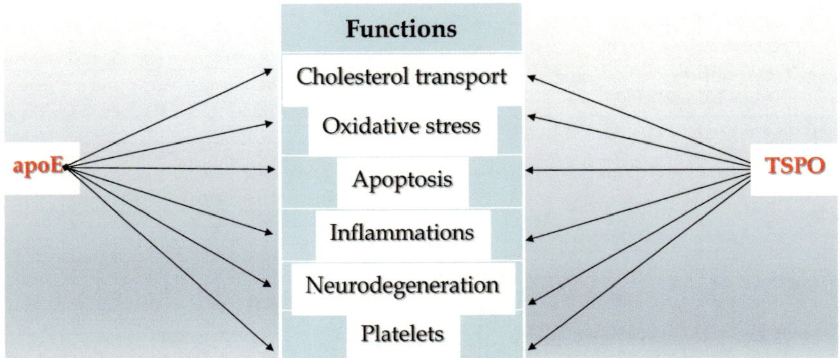

Figure 2. Possible correlations between Apo E and TSPO due to potential participation in various functions.

2. Materials and methods

Apolipoprotein E–deficient mice (Apo E KO mice) present a well-established model to study atherogenesis. In these mice, reverse cholesterol transport is dysfunctional, increasing the blood cholesterol level up to five times higher than in normal mice [66]. As Apo E deficiency causes increased cholesterol levels, which in turn may modulate TSPO function, we were interested to study whether TSPO binding characteristics may be affected in erythrocyte and platelet membranes. For this purpose, we used 12- to 14-week-old healthy male C57BL/6 mice (i.e. wild type, WT) and 14-week-old Apo E knockout (KO) mice. The mice were housed in polycarbonate cages in a pathogen-free facility set on a 12-h light–dark cycle and given *ad libitum* access to water and standard laboratory feed. All experimental procedures were carried out following the guidelines of the International European ethical standards for the care and use of laboratory animals (Community Council Directive 86-609). All protocols were approved and reviewed by the local ethics committee.

Platelets and erythrocytes preparation. Up to 1 mL of mouse blood was drawn by cardiac puncture of deeply anesthetized fasting mice in a terminal procedure and collected in plastic tubes containing trisodium citrate [3/8%, 1/10 (v:v)].

Platelet preparation

i. To obtain platelet-rich plasma (PRP), blood was centrifuged at 200×*g* for 20 min

ii. Then, 3/4 of the supernatant was collected to a new tube and centrifuged at 1000×*g* for 30 min

iii. The pellet was washed with Tyrode's buffer (Sigma-Aldrich, T1788) in a volume identical to the volume of the original fluid and centrifuged at 1000×*g* for 15 min and the pellet that contained only platelets was used for binding assay

Erythrocyte preparation

http://dx.doi.org/10.5772/61971

i. The pellet obtained from the first centrifugation (protocol i) at 200×*g*, was washed three times in isotonic solution of sodium chloride and used for isolation of erythrocyte membranes

ii. Purified erythrocytes were suspended in a 30-fold volume of 20 mM PBS containing 1 mM MgCl2, pH 7.5, allowed to stand for one hour prior to centrifugation at 13,000×*g*, 40 min at 4°C, in order to obtain erythrocyte membrane as pellet [67]

iii. Protein concentration of membrane preparations were determined by the Bradford assay [68, 69]

Assays of TSPO binding characteristics by [^{3}H]PK 11195 binding measurements. Maximal binding capacity (B_{max}) and equilibrium dissociation constant (K_d) of the binding of the TSPO-specific ligand, [^{3}H]PK 11195, in whole cell membrane preparations from the platelets and erythrocytes were assayed as described previously [40, 70, 71]. [^{3}H]PK 11195 (1-(2-chlorphenyl)-*N*-methyl-*N*-(1-methypropyl)-3-isoquinolinecarboxamide) was obtained from New England Nuclear (Boston, MA). Unlabeled PK 11195 was purchased from Sigma-Aldrich, Israel (Rehovot, Israel).

Procedure

- For binding assays of the B_{max} and the K_d, the reaction mixtures contained 400 μL of the membrane preparation in question (≈100 μg protein) and 25 μL of [^{3}H]PK 11195 solution (0.2 to 6 nM final concentrations) in the absence (total binding) or presence (nonspecific binding) of 75 μL unlabeled PK 11195 (10 μM final concentration)
- After incubation for 90 min in ice-water bath, the samples were vacuum filtered through Whatman GF/C filters, washed three times with 4 mL of 50 mM phosphate buffer and placed in vials containing 4 mL of Opti-Fluor (Waltham, MA)
- Radioactivity was counted after 12 h with a 1600CA Tri-Carb liquid scintillation analyser (Packard, Meriden, CT). Scatchard analysis of [^{3}H]PK 11195 binding was done to determine the B_{max} and K_d values
- For one point binding analysis, the concentration of 6 nM [^{3}H] PK 11195 was applied

The Bradford assay is based on the equilibrium between three forms of Coomassie blue G dye. Under strong acidic conditions, the dye is stable as a doubly protonated red form. Upon binding to protein, it is most stable as an unprotonated, blue form. Determination of microgram quantities of protein in the Bradford Coomassie brilliant blue assay is established by measurement of absorbance at 590 nm [69]. For this protein assay, Bradford solution (comprising Coomassie Brilliant Blue G-250 and an acid with a pKa of 1–2) was obtained from Bio-Rad (Munich, Germany).

Procedure

- 10 μL from each sample was mixed with 200 μL of Bradford solution in 96-well plates, and incubated for 10 min in the dark at room temperature

- Absorption was measured using an ELISA Reader or "ULTRASPECTRO 2000" at 595 nm. The protein concentration was determined by comparing the absorption values of the protein samples to the appropriate BSA standard curve, prepared from the BSA volumes: 0, 2, 4, 8, 10, 15, 20, 25, 50, 100 and 150 μL, completed to a final volume of 800 μL by DDW

3. Results with discussion

Atherosclerosis is characterized by inflammatory infiltration into the arterial wall of macrophages, dendritic cells, platelets and activated T cells, resulting in plaque formation. This process is initiated by inappropriate lipid metabolism, calcium signaling and increased burden of secretory pathways [3]. Macrophages, especially in the atherosclerotic plaque, contribute to the local inflammatory responses by secreting proinflammatory cytokines [72]. Activated macrophages have been demonstrated with high TSPO expression levels [73, 74]. TSPO has been identified in human leukocytes and erythrocytes and appears to play roles in several aspects of the immune response and the regulation of the host defense response in general [43, 46]. In addition, TSPO was detected in the plasma membrane of neutrophils, where it was shown to stimulate adhesion and motility [75].

Apolipoprotein E may also be involved in the immune response, as suggested by the impaired immune response in Apo E-deficient mice [76]. TSPO levels in platelets of rats and humans have been demonstrated to respond to a wide variety of pathological conditions [46, 77, 78]. It has been suggested that TSPO density in platelets can be used as a promising biological marker of stressful conditions [79–81].

To determine TSPO binding characteristics in Apo E-KO mice, we applied binding assays with the TSPO-specific ligand [^{3}H] PK 11195. Since cholesterol plays an important role in steroidogenesis, atherosclerosis and Alzheimer's disease, which have been correlated with TSPO and Apo E expression, we expected to find changes in TSPO binding levels in platelets and erythrocytes of Apo E-knockout mice compared to their WT strain. Indeed, regarding the platelets and erythrocytes, a significant increase ($p < 0.05$) in TSPO binding was noticed in Apo E knockout mice compared to WT (Table 1). In addition, our results showed no major difference in TSPO B_{max} between WT and Apo E-KO mice in other tissues (data not shown); suggesting that the effects seen on platelets and erythrocytes may be quite specific in relation to atherosclerosis.

Scatchard analysis demonstrates [^{3}H]PK 11195 binding of 1923 ± 1010 fmol/mg protein in erythrocyte membranes of wild-type mice vs. 3142 ± 1761 fmol/mg measured in erythrocytes membranes in the Apo E KO group (Figure 2). The obtained results from erythrocytes' membranes in our study are in the range of those in human membranes as measured by Olson et al. [67]. In these human erythrocytes, the B_{max} was 1120 fmol/mg protein and the K_d 3.9 ± 0.4 nM. It has been suggested that TSPO present in the plasma membrane of erythrocytes is involved in redistribution of intracellular cholesterol to change the nuclear membrane rigidity prior to erythrocyte maturation [82]. Recent studies by us have shown that TSPO is involved in the regulation of gene expression as well as heme metabolism [45, 83, 84]. More studies may provide deeper insights into how TSPO is involved in molecular biological mechanisms and biological functions of erythrocytes.

	Wild type mice			Apo E KO mice		
Cells	B/6nM (fmoles/mg)	Kd (nM)	n	B/6nM (fmoles/mg)	Kd (nM)	n
Platelets	1445 ± 736	0.8 ± 0.3	6	**6201 ± 2681****	1.3 ± 0.5	6
Erythrocytes	1923 ± 1010	2.6 ± 0.8	7	**3142 ± 1761***	4.2 ± 1.8	6

Table 1. [^{3}H] PK 11195 binding parameters in mice erythrocyte and platelet membranes

Average B values fmoles/mg protein and K_d values (nM) of 6 nM [^{3}H]PK 11195 binding to TSPO in erythrocyte and platelets membranes of WT (Bb-Control) and Apo E KO mice, fed with standard feed. One-way analysis of variance ANOVA was used, with Mann–Whitney as the post hoc, nonparametric test. Data are expressed as mean ± SD; *, $p < 0.05$; **, $p < 0.01$, vs. control.

Activated platelets are detected in increased numbers in the circulation of patients with atherosclerosis, coronary artery disease, and hypercholesterolemia. In the advanced atherosclerosis model of Apo E KO mice, subendothelial infiltration of monocytes/macrophages and platelets was observed, suggesting intimate interactions of platelets and macrophages in early atherosclerosis [85]. A recent paper by Nishikawa et al. demonstrated the role of hydrogen sulfide (H_2S), a gasotransmitter, in inhibiting platelet aggregation by interfering the cytosolic Ca^{2+} mobilization in a cAMP-dependent manner, comparable to what is observed for nitric oxide (NO) [86]. Studies by us have suggested that functions regulated by NO require the presence and activation of TSPO [87]. A study from Hamilton et al. indicated that activation of platelets with thrombin and other agents can promote atherogenesis [2]. Activation of human platelets is inhibited by two intracellular pathways regulated by either cyclic AMP or cyclic GMP. The importance of cyclic second messengers in modulating platelet reactivity is well established, elaborating the lipid-lowering effects of simvastatin therapy on inhibition of platelet aggregation through increasing the levels of both cAMP and cGMP [4]. Although Apo E induced increases in both cAMP and cGMP, additional experiments implicated a specific stimulation of guanylate cyclase activity and a rise in cGMP as prerequisites for the inhibitory effects on platelet aggregation of Apo E. Nonetheless, the mechanisms by which platelets promote atherogenesis need further observations.

Both TSPO and Apo E have been found to be involved in neurodegeneration. Both molecules have been associated with particular common factors being part of neurodegenerative diseases, such as cholesterol metabolism, oxidative stress, apoptosis and inflammation (Figure 1). Furthermore, Apo E was found to be involved in platelet aggregation, while TSPO expression in platelets has been associated with various pathological conditions, including neurological disorders [46]. Some authors have reported the protective effects of TSPO agonists in

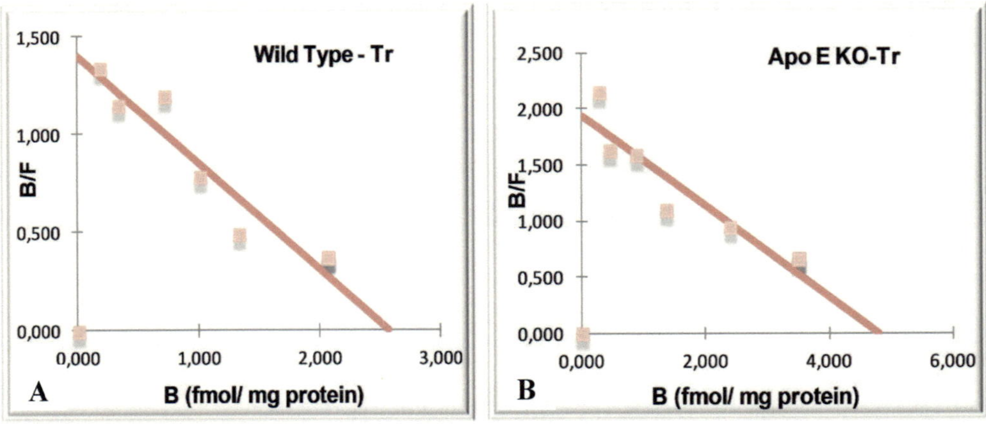

Figure 3. Representative examples of Scatchard plots of saturation curves of [^{3}H] PK 11195 binding to membrane preparations of platelets of wild-type mice (A) and apo E-KO mice (B). Abbreviations: B, bound; B/F, bound over free.

experimental neuropathy, suggesting reparative actions of brain TSPO in such a disease [88]. A recent study from Giannaccini et al. demonstrated upregulated TSPO expression in the brain region of leptin-deficient obese mice (ob/ob) [89]. In addition, the induction of TSPO expression under neuropathological conditions suggests that this molecule may be involved in the response of the neural tissue to inflammation [90, 91]. Indeed, application of TSPO ligands can dramatically decrease neuropathological symptoms of various diseases and injuries [61, 62]. However, the precise role of TSPO in the injured neural tissue needs to be investigated further.

In conclusion, the platelets' and erythrocytes' constant exposure to enhanced levels of cholesterol in the bloodstream may be associated with increased TSPO levels. One mechanism may be that apoE's modulation of NO levels may affect TSPO expression in the platelets and erythrocytes. Our study indicates that the Apo E mouse presents a promising animal model to elucidate the exact role of TSPO in platelets and erythrocytes in a cholesterol-dependent atherosclerosis. Thus, the TSPO represent a novel therapeutic target and diagnostic tool for cardiovascular disease and its complications.

Explanation of abbreviations and symbols: ANOVA, analysis of variance; ApoE$^{-/-}$ KO, apolipoprotein E knockout mice; ApoER, apolipoprotein E receptor; BSA, bovine serum albumin; cAMP, adenosine 3,5-cyclic monophosphate; DBI, diazepam binding inhibitor; CAM, cell adhesion molecule; Er, erythrocytes; H_2S, hydrogen sulfide; HDL, high-density lipoprotein; kDa, kilodalton; K_d, equilibrium dissociation constant; K_m, equilibrium constant related to Michaelis–Menten kinetics (similarly, K_d, K_a, K_{eq}, K_s); LDL, low-density lipoproteins; LDLR, low-density lipoprotein receptor; LOX-1, the lectin-like endothelial receptor for ox-LDL; mPTP, mitochondrial permeability transition pore; MCP-1, monocyte chemoattractant protein-1; NADP, nicotinamide adenine dinucleotide phosphate; NADH, reduced nicotinamide adenine dinucleotide; NO, nitric oxide; NOS, nitric oxide synthase; ox-LDL, oxidized low-density lipoproteins; PBR, peripheral-type benzodiazepine receptor; PK 11195, 1-(2-

chlorophenyl)-N-methyl-N-(1-methyl-prop1)-3 isoquinoline carboxamide; ROS, reactive oxygen species; TSPO, 18 kDa translocator protein.

Author details

Jasmina Dimitrova-Shumkovska[1 #], Leo Veenman[2 #], Inbar Roim[2], Svetlana Leschiner[2] and Moshe Gavish[2*]

*Address all correspondence to: mgavish@tx.technion.ac.i

1 Department of Experimental Biochemistry and Physiology, Faculty of Natural Sciences and Mathematics, Institute of Biology, Ss. Cyril and Methodius University, Skopje, Republic of Macedonia

2 Department of Molecular Pharmacology, Rappaport Family Institute for Research in the Medical Sciences, Technion-Israel Institute of Technology, Haifa, Israel

Author Contributions: Jasmina Dimitrova-Shumkovska and Leo Veenman contributed equally to this book chapter.

References

[1] Camici PG, Rimoldi OE, Gaemperli O, Libby P. Non-invasive anatomic and functional imaging of vascular inflammation and unstable plaque. Eur Heart J 2012; 33:1309–1317.

[2] Hamilton JR, Cornelissen I, Mountford JK, Coughlin SR. Atherosclerosis proceeds independently of thrombin-induced platelet activation in ApoE$^{-/-}$ mice. Atherosclerosis 2009; 205:427–432.

[3] Li H, Horke S, Forstermann U. Vascular oxidative stress, nitric oxide and atherosclerosis. Atherosclerosis 2014; 237:208–219.

[4] Lee YM, Chen WF, Chou DS, et al. Cyclic nucleotides and mitogen-activated protein kinases: regulation of simvastatin in platelet activation. J Biomed Sci 2010; 17:45.

[5] West LE, Steiner T, Judge HM, Francis SE, Storey RF. Vessel wall, not platelet, P2Y12 potentiates early atherogenesis. Cardiovasc Res 2014; 102:429–435.

[6] Kolodgie FD, Gold HK, Burke AP, et al. Intraplaque hemorrhage and progression of coronary atheroma. N Engl J Med 2003; 349:2316–2325.

[7] Bultmann A, Li Z, Wagner S, et al. Impact of glycoprotein VI and platelet adhesion on atherosclerosis—a possible role of fibronectin. J Mol Cell Cardiol 2010; 49:532–542.

[8] Massberg S, Brand K, Gruner S, et al. A critical role of platelet adhesion in the initiation of atherosclerotic lesion formation. J Exp Med 2002; 196:887–896.

[9] Gonzalez J, Donoso W, Diaz N, et al. High fat diet induces adhesion of platelets to endothelium in two models of dyslipidemia. J Obes 2014; 2014:591270.

[10] Carnevale R, Bartimoccia S, Nocella C, et al. LDL oxidation by platelets propagates platelet activation via an oxidative stress-mediated mechanism. Atherosclerosis 2014; 237:108–116.

[11] Chen Y, Cai T, Wang H, et al. Regulation of intracellular cholesterol distribution by Na/K-ATPase. J Biol Chem 2009; 284:14881–14890.

[12] Mehta RL, Kellum JA, Shah SV, et al. Acute Kidney Injury Network: report of an initiative to improve outcomes in acute kidney injury. Crit Care 2007; 11:R31.

[13] Podrez EA, Byzova TV, Febbraio M, et al. Platelet CD36 links hyperlipidemia, oxidant stress and a prothrombotic phenotype. Nat Med 2007; 13:1086–1095.

[14] Pirillo A, Norata GD, Catapano AL. LOX-1, OxLDL, and atherosclerosis. Mediators Inflamm 2013; 2013:152786.

[15] Yoshimoto R, Fujita Y, Kakino A, Iwamoto S, Takaya T, Sawamura T. The discovery of LOX-1, its ligands and clinical significance. Cardiovasc Drugs Ther 2011; 25:379–391.

[16] Elliott DA, Kim WS, Jans DA, Garner B. Macrophage apolipoprotein-E knockdown modulates caspase-3 activation without altering sensitivity to apoptosis. Biochim Biophys Acta 2008; 1780:145–153.

[17] Quinn CM, Kagedal K, Terman A, et al. Induction of fibroblast apolipoprotein E expression during apoptosis, starvation-induced growth arrest and mitosis. Biochem J 2004; 378:753–761.

[18] Mahley RW, Weisgraber KH, Innerarity TL. Interaction of plasma lipoproteins containing apolipoproteins B and E with heparin and cell surface receptors. Biochim Biophys Acta 1979; 575:81–91.

[19] Gianturco SH, Gotto AM, Jr., Hwang SL, et al. Apolipoprotein E mediates uptake of Sf 100–400 hypertriglyceridemic very low density lipoproteins by the low density lipoprotein receptor pathway in normal human fibroblasts. J Biol Chem 1983; 258:4526–4533.

[20] Hussain MM, Mahley RW, Boyles JK, Fainaru M, Brecht WJ, Lindquist PA. Chylomicron-chylomicron remnant clearance by liver and bone marrow in rabbits. Factors that modify tissue-specific uptake. J Biol Chem 1989; 264:9571–9582.

[21] Mahley RW. Apolipoprotein E: cholesterol transport protein with expanding role in cell biology. Science 1988; 240:622–630.

http://dx.doi.org/10.5772/61971

[22] Bird JL, Izquierdo-Garcia D, Davies JR, et al. Evaluation of translocator protein quantification as a tool for characterising macrophage burden in human carotid atherosclerosis. Atherosclerosis 2010; 210:388–391.

[23] Linton MF, Fazio S. Macrophages, lipoprotein metabolism, and atherosclerosis: insights from murine bone marrow transplantation studies. Curr Opin Lipidol 1999; 10:97–105.

[24] Bellosta S, Nathan BP, Orth M, Dong LM, Mahley RW, Pitas RE. Stable expression and secretion of apolipoproteins E3 and E4 in mouse neuroblastoma cells produces differential effects on neurite outgrowth. J Biol Chem 1995; 270:27063–27071.

[25] Kashyap VS, Santamarina-Fojo S, Brown DR, et al. Apolipoprotein E deficiency in mice: gene replacement and prevention of atherosclerosis using adenovirus vectors. J Clin Invest 1995; 96:1612–1620.

[26] Hansson GK, Edfeldt K. Toll to be paid at the gateway to the vessel wall. Arterioscler Thromb Vasc Biol 2005; 25:1085–1087.

[27] Ophir G, Amariglio N, Jacob-Hirsch J, Elkon R, Rechavi G, Michaelson DM. Apolipoprotein E4 enhances brain inflammation by modulation of the NF-kappaB signaling cascade. Neurobiol Dis 2005; 20:709–718.

[28] Zeiffer U, Schober A, Lietz M, et al. Neointimal smooth muscle cells display a proinflammatory phenotype resulting in increased leukocyte recruitment mediated by P-selectin and chemokines. Circ Res 2004; 94:776–784.

[29] Sjogren M, Blennow K. The link between cholesterol and Alzheimer's disease. World J Biol Psychiatry 2005; 6:85–97.

[30] Wang ZY, Miki T, Ding Y, et al. A high cholesterol diet given to apolipoprotein E-knockout mice has a differential effect on the various neurotrophin systems in the hippocampus. Metab Brain Dis 2011; 26:185–194.

[31] Masliah E, Mallory M, Ge N, Alford M, Veinbergs I, Roses AD. Neurodegeneration in the central nervous system of apoE-deficient mice. Exp Neurol 1995; 136:107–122.

[32] Poirier J. Apolipoprotein E in the brain and its role in Alzheimer's disease. J Psychiatry Neurosci 1996; 21:128–134.

[33] DeMattos RB, Curtiss LK, Williams DL. A minimally lipidated form of cell-derived apolipoprotein E exhibits isoform-specific stimulation of neurite outgrowth in the absence of exogenous lipids or lipoproteins. J Biol Chem 1998; 273:4206–4212.

[34] Marques MA, Tolar M, Harmony JA, Crutcher KA. A thrombin cleavage fragment of apolipoprotein E exhibits isoform-specific neurotoxicity. Neuroreport 1996; 7:2529–2532.

[35] Strittmatter WJ, Saunders AM, Schmechel D, et al. Apolipoprotein E: high-avidity binding to beta-amyloid and increased frequency of type 4 allele in late-onset familial Alzheimer disease. Proc Natl Acad Sci U S A 1993; 90:1977–1981.

[36] Riddell DR, Graham A, Owen JS. Apolipoprotein E inhibits platelet aggregation through the L-arginine:nitric oxide pathway. Implications for vascular disease. J Biol Chem 1997; 272:89–95.

[37] Heemskerk JW, Sage SO. Calcium signalling in platelets and other cells. Platelets 1994; 5:295–316.

[38] Smolenski A. Novel roles of cAMP/cGMP-dependent signaling in platelets. J Thromb Haemost 2012; 10:167–176.

[39] Dimitrova-Shumkovska J, Veenman L, Gavish M, The 18 kDa translocator protein as a potential participant in atherosclerosis, In "Atherogenesis": edited by Pathasarathy, S., ISBN 978-953-307-992-9, INTECH, 2012.

[40] Dimitrova-Shumkovska J, Veenman L, Ristoski T, Leschiner S, Gavish M. Chronic high fat, high cholesterol supplementation decreases 18 kDa translocator protein binding capacity in association with increased oxidative stress in rat liver and aorta. Food Chem Toxicol 2010; 48:910–921.

[41] Dimitrova-Shumkovska J, Veenman L, Roim I, Gavish M, The 18 kDa translocator protein and atherosclerosis in mice lacking apolipoprotein E, In "Lipid Metabolism": edited by Baez RV, ISBN 978-953-51-0944-0, INTECH, 2013: 91–118.

[42] Onyimba JA, Coronado MJ, Garton AE, et al. The innate immune response to coxsackievirus B3 predicts progression to cardiovascular disease and heart failure in male mice. Biol Sex Differ 2011; 2:2.

[43] Veenman L, Papadopoulos V, Gavish M. Channel-like functions of the 18-kDa translocator protein (TSPO): regulation of apoptosis and steroidogenesis as part of the host-defense response. Curr Pharm Des 2007; 13:2385–2405.

[44] Anholt RR, De Souza EB, Kuhar MJ, Snyder SH. Depletion of peripheral-type benzodiazepine receptors after hypophysectomy in rat adrenal gland and testis. Eur J Pharmacol 1985; 110:41–46.

[45] Zeno S, Veenman L, Katz Y, Bode J, Gavish M, Zaaroor M. The 18 kDa mitochondrial translocator protein (TSPO) prevents accumulation of protoporphyrin IX. Involvement of reactive oxygen species (ROS). Curr Mol Med 2012; 12:494–501.

[46] Veenman L, Gavish M. The peripheral-type benzodiazepine receptor and the cardiovascular system. Implications for drug development. Pharmacol Ther 2006; 110:503–524.

[47] Marshall JS, Jawdat DM. Mast cells in innate immunity. J Allergy Clin Immunol 2004; 114:21–27.

[48] Wojta J, Huber K, Valent P. New aspects in thrombotic research: complement induced switch in mast cells from a profibrinolytic to a prothrombotic phenotype. Pathophysiol Haemost Thromb 2003; 33:438–441.

[49] Lenfant M, Zavala F, Haumont J, Potier P. [Presence of a peripheral type benzodiazepine binding site on the macrophage; its possible role in immunomodulation]. C R Acad Sci III 1985; 300:309–314.

[50] Verma A, Nye JS, Snyder SH. Porphyrins are endogenous ligands for the mitochondrial (peripheral-type) benzodiazepine receptor. Proc Natl Acad Sci U S A 1987; 84:2256–2260.

[51] Caballero B, Veenman L, Gavish M. Role of mitochondrial translocator protein (18 kDa) on mitochondrial- related cell death processes. Recent Pat Endocr Metab Immune Drug Discov 2013; 7:86–101.

[52] Jaremko L, Jaremko M, Giller K, Becker S, Zweckstetter M. Structure of the mitochondrial translocator protein in complex with a diagnostic ligand. Science 2014; 343:1363–1366.

[53] Kim EJ, Yu SW. Translocator protein 18 kDa (TSPO): old dogma, new mice, new structure, and new questions for neuroprotection. Neural Regen Res 2015; 10:878–880.

[54] Kugler W, Veenman L, Shandalov Y, et al. Ligands of the mitochondrial 18 kDa translocator protein attenuate apoptosis of human glioblastoma cells exposed to erucylphosphohomocholine. Cell Oncol 2008; 30:435–450.

[55] Levin E, Premkumar A, Veenman L, et al. The peripheral-type benzodiazepine receptor and tumorigenicity: isoquinoline binding protein (IBP) antisense knockdown in the C6 glioma cell line. Biochemistry 2005; 44:9924–9935.

[56] Midzak A, Akula N, Lecanu L, Papadopoulos V. Novel androstenetriol interacts with the mitochondrial translocator protein and controls steroidogenesis. J Biol Chem 2011; 286:9875–9887.

[57] Qi X, Xu J, Wang F, Xiao J. Translocator protein (18 kDa): a promising therapeutic target and diagnostic tool for cardiovascular diseases. Oxid Med Cell Longev 2012; 2012:162934.

[58] Veenman L, Gavish M, Kugler W. Apoptosis induction by erucylphosphohomocholine via the 18 kDa mitochondrial translocator protein: implications for cancer treatment. Anticancer Agents Med Chem 2014; 14:559–577.

[59] Waterfield JD, McGeer EG, McGeer PL. The peripheral benzodiazepine receptor ligand PK 11195 inhibits arthritis in the MRL-lpr mouse model. Rheumatology (Oxford) 1999; 38:1068–1073.

[60] Zeno S, Zaaroor M, Leschiner S, Veenman L, Gavish M. CoCl(2) induces apoptosis via the 18 kDa translocator protein in U118MG human glioblastoma cells. Biochemistry 2009; 48:4652–4661.

[61] Veenman L, Vainshtein A, Gavish M. TSPO as a target for treatments of diseases, including neuropathological disorders. Cell Death Dis 2015.

[62] Vainshtein A, Veenman L, Shterenberg A, et al. Quinazoline-based tricyclic compounds that regulate programmed cell death, induce neuronal differentiation, and are curative in animal models for excitotoxicity and hereditary brain disease. Cell Death Discovery 2015; 1.

[63] Veiga S, Carrero P, Pernia O, Azcoitia I, Garcia-Segura LM. Translocator protein 18 kDa is involved in the regulation of reactive gliosis. Glia 2007; 55:1426–1436.

[64] Torres SR, Frode TS, Nardi GM, et al. Anti-inflammatory effects of peripheral benzodiazepine receptor ligands in two mouse models of inflammation. Eur J Pharmacol 2000; 408:199–211.

[65] Bribes E, Bourrie B, Casellas P. Ligands of the peripheral benzodiazepine receptor have therapeutic effects in pneumopathies in vivo. Immunol Lett 2003; 88:241–247.

[66] Meir KS, Leitersdorf E. Atherosclerosis in the apolipoprotein-E-deficient mouse: a decade of progress. Arterioscler Thromb Vasc Biol 2004; 24:1006–1014.

[67] Olson JM, Ciliax BJ, Mancini WR, Young AB. Presence of peripheral-type benzodiazepine binding sites on human erythrocyte membranes. Eur J Pharmacol 1988; 152:47–53.

[68] Bradford MM. A rapid and sensitive method for the quantitation of microgram quantities of protein utilizing the principle of protein-dye binding. Anal Biochem 1976; 72:248–254.

[69] Zor T, Selinger Z. Linearization of the Bradford protein assay increases its sensitivity: theoretical and experimental studies. Anal Biochem 1996; 236:302–308.

[70] Awad M, Gavish M. Solubilization of peripheral-type benzodiazepine binding sites from cat cerebral cortex. J Neurochem 1989; 52:1880–1885.

[71] Danovich L, Veenman L, Leschiner S, et al. The influence of clozapine treatment and other antipsychotics on the 18 kDa translocator protein, formerly named the peripheral-type benzodiazepine receptor, and steroid production. Eur Neuropsychopharmacol 2008; 18:24–33.

[72] Goldstein JL, Brown MS. The LDL receptor. Arterioscler, Thromb Vasc Biol 2009; 29:431–438.

[73] Fujimura Y, Hwang PM, Trout Iii H, et al. Increased peripheral benzodiazepine receptors in arterial plaque of patients with atherosclerosis: an autoradiographic study with [(3)H]PK 11195. Atherosclerosis 2008; 201:108–111.

[74] Gaemperli O, Shalhoub J, Owen DR, et al. Imaging intraplaque inflammation in carotid atherosclerosis with 11C-PK11195 positron emission tomography/computed tomography. Eur Heart J 2012; 33:1902–1910.

[75] de Lima CB, Tamura EK, Montero-Melendez T, et al. Actions of translocator protein ligands on neutrophil adhesion and motility induced by G-protein coupled receptor signaling. Biochem Biophys Res Commun 2012; 417:918–923.

[76] de Bont N, Netea MG, Demacker PN, Kullberg BJ, van der Meer JW, Stalenhoef AF. Apolipoprotein E-deficient mice have an impaired immune response to *Klebsiella pneumoniae*. Eur J Clin Invest 2000; 30:818–822.

[77] Benavides J, Malgouris C, Imbault F, et al. "Peripheral type" benzodiazepine binding sites in rat adrenals: binding studies with [3H]PK 11195 and autoradiographic localization. Arch Int Pharmacodyn Ther 1983; 266:38–49.

[78] Canat X, Guillaumont A, Bouaboula M, et al. Peripheral benzodiazepine receptor modulation with phagocyte differentiation. Biochem Pharmacol 1993; 46:551–554.

[79] Gavish M, Bachman I, Shoukrun R, et al. Enigma of the peripheral benzodiazepine receptor. Pharmacol Rev 1999; 51:629–650.

[80] Martini C, Chelli B, Betti L, et al. Peripheral benzodiazepine binding sites in platelets of patients affected by mitochondrial diseases and large scale mitochondrial DNA rearrangements. Mol Med 2002; 8:841–846.

[81] Nakamura K, Fukunishi I, Nakamoto Y, Iwahashi K, Yoshii M. Peripheral-type benzodiazepine receptors on platelets are correlated with the degrees of anxiety in normal human subjects. Psychopharmacology 2002; 162:301–303.

[82] Fan J, Rone MB, Papadopoulos V. Translocator protein 2 is involved in cholesterol redistribution during erythropoiesis. J Biol Chem 2009; 284:30484–30497.

[83] Bode J, Veenman L, Vainshtein A, Kugler W, Rosenberg BJ, Gavish M. Modulation of gene expression associated with the cell cycle and tumorigenicity of glioblastoma cells by the 18 kDa translocator protein (TSPO). Austin J Pharmacol Ther 2014; 2.

[84] Veenman L, Bode J, Gaitner M, et al. Effects of 18-kDa translocator protein knockdown on gene expression of glutamate receptors, transporters, and metabolism, and on cell viability affected by glutamate. Pharmacogenet Genomics 2012; 22:606–619.

[85] Stivala S, Reiner MF, Lohmann C, Luscher TF, Matter CM, Beer JH. Dietary alpha-linolenic acid increases the platelet count in ApoE$^{-/-}$ mice by reducing clearance. Blood 2013; 122:1026–1033.

[86] Nishikawa H, Hayashi H, Kubo S, Tsubota-Matsunami M, Sekiguchi F, Kawabata A. Inhibition by hydrogen sulfide of rabbit platelet aggregation and calcium mobilization. Biol Pharm Bull 2013; 36:1278–1282.

[87] Shargorodsky L, Veenman L, Caballero B, et al. The nitric oxide donor sodium nitroprusside requires the 18 kDa translocator protein to induce cell death. Apoptosis 2012; 17:647–665.

[88] Giatti S, Pesaresi M, Cavaletti G, et al. Neuroprotective effects of a ligand of translocator protein-18 kDa (Ro5-4864) in experimental diabetic neuropathy. Neuroscience 2009; 164:520–529.

[89] Giannaccini G, Betti L, Palego L, et al. Serotonin transporter (SERT) and translocator protein (TSPO) expression in the obese ob/ob mouse. BMC Neurosci 2011; 12:18.

[90] Papadopoulos V, Lecanu L. Translocator protein (18 kDa) TSPO: an emerging therapeutic target in neurotrauma. Exp Neurol 2009; 219:53–57.

[91] Veenman L, Gavish M. Peripheral-type benzodiazepine receptors: their implication in brain disease. Drug Development Research 2000; 50:355–370.

Chapter 4

Is Restenosis/Reocclusion after Femoropopliteal Percutaneous Transluminal Angioplasty (PTA) the Consequence of Reduced Blood Flow, Inflammation, and/or Hemostasis Disturbances?

Mojca Božič-Mijovski, Vinko Boc, Vladka Salapura, Aleš Blinc and Mojca Stegnar

Additional information is available at the end of the chapter

http://dx.doi.org/10.5772/61519

Abstract

Percutaneous transluminal angioplasty (PTA) is an established method for treatment of peripheral artery disease (PAD) of the femoropopliteal artery. However, in up to 50% of patients restenosis and/or reocclusion remain a frequent complication occurring in the first year after the procedure. In this study, we focused on the influence of compromised postprocedural infrapopliteal runoff of the affected limb, on the hypercoagulability as detected by a global hemostasis assay and on genetic predisposition to hypercoagulability and on the regulation of the inflammation through the nuclear receptor related 1 protein (NuRR1). Consecutive PAD patients treated by femoropopliteal PTA because of disabling claudication or critical limb ischemia were followed up by vascular ultrasound imaging at 1, 6, and 12 months after the procedure. Venous blood samples for hemostasis, inflammation, and gene analysis were obtained before and 24 h after PTA. One month after femoropopliteal PTA, 23% of patients with compromised runoff developed the combined end point restenosis/reocclusion in comparison to 11% with good runoff ($p = 0.03$). After 6 months, the differences were no longer significant. It was concluded that compromised postprocedural infrapopliteal runoff predisposes to early restenosis/reocclusion after femoropopliteal PTA and that the deterioration of infrapopliteal runoff in the year after femoropopliteal PTA is accompanied by worsening of long-term femoropopliteal patency. Patients were genotyped for the prothrombotic gene polymorphisms: platelet receptor glycoprotein IIIa T1565C, coagulation factor V G1691A, coagulation factor II G20210A, coagulation factor XII C(-4)T, and plasminogen activator inhibitor-1 4G5G. We were not able to show any association between these polymorphisms and the restenosis/reocclusion rate in patients treated with femoropopliteal PTA. Furthermore, no association between thrombin generation and restenosis/reocclusion rate was established. NuRR1 haplotypes significantly increased the restenosis/reocclusion rate after PTA (adjusted relative risks were 1.6, 95% CI 1.1–2.3 for haplotype 2 and 2.0, 95% CI 1.3–2.8 for haplotype 3). To conclude, this study suggested a significantly higher restenosis/reocclusion rate in patients with compromised runoff compared to patients with a good runoff 1 month after the procedure. Hypercoagulability was not associated with the restenosis/reocclusion rate, and the prothrombotic polymorphisms were equally distributed among patient with and without restenosis/reocclusion, suggesting minor or no role in restenosis/reocclusion. Haplotypes 2 and 3 in the NuRR1 gene significantly increased the restenosis/reocclusion rate, suggesting significant role of inflammation. In this ongoing study, further analysis on a larger group of patients is warranted.

Keywords: Percutaneous transluminal angioplasty, peripheral artery disease, inflammation, hemostasis

1. Introduction

Peripheral artery disease (PAD) is a prevalent circulatory problem in which narrowed or occluded arteries reduce blood flow to the limbs. PAD is most often a manifestation of generalized atherosclerosis that reduces the patients' quality of life by reducing their walking ability and also confers an increased risk for cardiac death, acute coronary syndrome, and ischemic stroke. Patients with PAD die more than 3 times more often than peers of the same age [1]. Early diagnosis is important for improving the patient's quality of life and for reducing the risk of serious secondary vascular events. PAD, defined by decreased ankle brachial pressure index, is found in 15–20% of population aged 55 years or more [2]. All patients with PAD require preventive treatment against vascular events by lifestyle modification and protective medication, but only a fraction ever requires a revascularization procedure [3, 4]. This procedure is needed in order to establish suitable blood flow to the affected limb if PAD severely hampers walking ability or in cases of critical limb ischemia [3, 4]. Percutaneous transluminal angioplasty (PTA) is an established revascularization method for treatment of PAD and is associated with low morbidity and mortality rates [3, 4]. However, in up to 60% of patients, restenosis and/or reocclusion remain a frequent complication occurring in the first year after the procedure [5]. Our understanding of the mechanisms of restenosis/reocclusion of the femoral artery after PTA is incomplete. The comprehension of the factors that contribute to the pathophysiology of restenosis/reocclusion is the foundation to develop effective strategies for improvement of patients' post-PTA outcome. Once identified, reliable predictors of the restenosis/reocclusion risk could facilitate the use of preventive measures, help to save healthcare resources, and assist in new drug development. In this study, we focused (i) on the influence of compromised postprocedural infrapopliteal runoff of the affected limb, (ii) on the hypercoagulability as detected by a global hemostasis assay and on genetic predisposition to hypercoagulability due to altered hemostatic factors that could support thrombus formation in the arterial segment injured by PTA, and (iii) on the regulation of the inflammation through

http://dx.doi.org/10.5772/61519

the nuclear receptor related 1 protein (NuRR1) that could presumable favor increased restenosis/reocclusion rate after successful PTA.

2. Problem statement

PAD causes inadequate blood flow to the limbs, mostly lower limbs. Femoropopliteal artery is the most commonly affected arterial segment. The patency of femoropopliteal artery after PTA is affected by several factors [37], including clinical severity of PAD, patient comorbidities, such as diabetes or renal failure, morphological characteristics of the arterial lesions, i.e., occlusion vs. stenosis, length of the lesion and their number, calcification of plaques, functional characteristics of the affected artery, i.e., the extent of vascular inflammation, and hemodynamic conditions that are to a large extent defined by the arterial runoff.

The STAR registry and several older studies listed poor tibial runoff as strongly predictive of bad long-term patency [6–10], but some authors found no association of femoral artery patency with tibial runoff 1 year after recanalization [11]. There is not much data on the role of concomitant infrapopliteal PTA in maintaining the long-term patency of the femoropopliteal segment after PTA. This question is difficult to address directly since it is not ethically acceptable to deny PTA of accessible lesions in the calf arteries to any group of patients with clinically relevant limb ischemia who are already treated by femoropopliteal PTA.

The acute response to arterial injury induced by PTA involves the adhesion of platelets and leukocytes, which react with the damaged arterial wall in proportion to the degree of injury. In addition, arterial injury activates hemostasis presumably, resulting in thrombus formation on the injured vessel segment [12]. The laboratory recognition of activated hemostasis (hypercoagulability) is a very demanding task due to the complexity of the hemostatic system. Hypercoagulability can be detected by global tests, such as the thrombin generation assay that provide an overview of the entire hemostatic system, including enzymes, cofactors, and inhibitors. With this assay hypercoagulability was detected in patients with atherothrombosis [13]. Another approach to detect hypercoagulability is to measure specific substances (peptides, enzymes, and enzyme–inhibitor complexes) that are liberated with the activation of hemostasis, namely, specific hemostasis activation markers such as D-dimer [14]. A permanent prothrombotic state caused by gene polymorphisms that affect coagulation factors or platelets could supplement hypercoagulability and contribute to increased risk for restenosis/reocclusion. Such prothrombotic polymorphisms include glycoprotein IIIa T1565C polymorphism (GPIIIa T1565C), which increases platelet adhesion and aggregation, factor V G1691A, which causes resistance to activated protein C, factor II G20210A associated with elevated prothrombin levels, factor XII C46T associated with lower factor XII levels, and plasminogen activator inhibitor-1 (PAI-1) 4G5G associated with lower PAI-1 levels.

In the following months after PTA, the hyperplasia of smooth muscle cells (SMCs) in vascular wall that is regulated by proinflammatory mediators can lead to restenosis [12, 15]. The association between inflammation and PAD is well established, and the prognostic value of inflammation in restenosis has also been recognized [16]. Shear stress during balloon inflation and vascular injury stimulates the production of proinflammatory molecules and the activation of circulating monocytes. The level of monocyte activation and adherence to the vascular wall, mediated by selectins and adhesion molecules, was suggested to promote late lumen loss [17]. The regulation of the inflammation through the nuclear receptor related 1 protein (NuRR1) has recently been associated with restenosis. NuRR1 (or NR4A2) together with NR4A1 and NR4A3 constitutes the nuclear receptor subfamily 4, group A (NR4A). This subfamily is also referred to as the nerve growth factor-induced protein-B subfamily of nuclear receptors because these receptors were first described as early response transcription factors expressed following stimulation by growth factors. All three subfamily members bind the same response element(s). They are referred to as orphan receptors because the ligands that may regulate their transcriptional activity have not yet been identified. These transcriptional factors have been described in the regulation of differentiation, proliferation, apoptosis, and survival of many different cell types [18]. Besides direct binding to the promoter of target genes, NuRR1 modulates gene transcription by the transrepression of other transcription factors. Its role in inflammatory responses has been recognized when the overexpression of NuRR1 in human atherosclerotic lesions compared to normal healthy human arteries has been observed [19]. An antiproliferative and anti-inflammatory function of NuRR1 in human SMCs and its protective role against arterial wall injury-induced SMC-rich lesion formation in mice has been shown [20]. The NuRR1 gene lies in one linkage disequilibrium block spanning approximately 36 kb of DNA on chromosome 2q22–2q23. Several gene polymorphisms were described in the NuRR1 gene; however, from the three tagging single-nucleotide polymorphisms (rs1466408, rs13428968, and rs12803), four haplotypes had been inferred with frequencies >1% that explained 96% of the variation in this linkage disequilibrium block [21]. In patients undergoing percutaneous coronary intervention, haplotypes 3 and 4 increased the risk of in-stent restenosis, target lesion revascularization, percutaneous coronary reinterventions, and the rate of major cardiac events (MACE) about 2- to 3-fold in the first year after the procedure [20]. A similar role in femoropopliteal restenosis after PTA was expected. To our knowledge, the role of NuRR1 haplotypes in femoropopliteal restenosis after PTA has not been investigated yet, although it could be expected.

3. Patients and methods

In our study on the effect of tibial runoff on femoropopliteal patency after PTA [22], consecutive consenting patients with claudication or critical limb ischemia admitted for femoropopliteal PTA to the Department of Vascular Diseases of the University Medical Centre Ljubljana have been enrolled and prospectively followed up. In addition to femoropopliteal PTA, infrapopliteal PTA has been performed in all cases when lesions of the calf arteries have been judged suitable for intervention. At enrolment, risk factors for PAD and clinical stage of PAD by the Fontaine classification have been determined for each patient [3]. The morphological changes of femoropopliteal lesions have been evaluated according to the TASC II classification [3]. Ankle brachial pressure index has been measured routinely before and after PTA [23]. The PTA procedures have been performed in a catheter laboratory by interventional radiologists.

The ipsilateral anterograde approach via the common femoral artery has been used except in cases of ostial lesions of the femoral artery, where the contralateral or transpopliteal approach has been used, introducing 5 Fr sheaths for vascular access. All patients, already treated with low-dose aspirin, have received local anesthesia and 3,000 IU heparin i.v. at the beginning of the procedure. Most stenotic lesions have been crossed by a soft 0.035-inch J-wire (Terumo Medical Corporation, USA) and in the majority of occlusions have been crossed by the direct recanalization technique. Alternatively, the subintimal approach has been used in cases of unsuccessful direct recanalization. Noncompliant balloons of 5 or 6 mm diameter from different manufacturers have been used, depending on the vessel diameter in the adjacent nondiseased parts. The balloons have been inflated for at least 1 min to 8 atm pressure. Stents (nitinol self-expanding stents) have been implanted only in cases of flow-limiting dissections or residual stenosis of >50% even after repeated balloon inflation. In patients with accessible concomitant infrapopliteal lesions, the PTA of the calf arteries has also been performed. For infrapopliteal lesions, 0.025-inch J-Terumo wire or 0.014/0.018-inch (Pointer, Denmark or Invatec, Italy) wires have been used for intraluminal crossing, with balloon diameters from 2 to 3.5 mm (different manufacturers). All angiographies have been performed by the standard digital subtraction technique. The technical success of PTA and the infrapopliteal runoff has been evaluated by periprocedural angiography. Immediate technical success has been defined as ≤ 50% residual angiographic stenosis [24]. Infrapopliteal runoff has been scored by a modification of the Society for Vascular Surgery criteria, originally intended for quantifying bypass runoff, where a higher score implies worse runoff [25]. This scoring system ascribes 3 points for occlusion throughout the vessel, 2.5 points for occlusion of less than half of the arterial length, 2 points for maximal stenosis of 50–99%, 1 point for maximal stenosis of 20–49%, and 0 points for less than 20% maximal stenosis. Each of the calf arteries has been ascribed a weight, i.e., multiplication factor, of 1, and the distal popliteal artery has been ascribed a weight of 3, with one point always added to the total score [26]. Thus, the cumulative score for the distal popliteal artery (a maximum of 9 + 1) and for the tibial vessels (a maximum of 3 × 3) gives a maximum score of 19 [23]. We have divided the patients' limbs into two categories: good runoff (<5 points) and compromised runoff (≥ 5 points). In the good runoff group, a limb has to have a patent popliteal artery and at least two patent calf arteries with less than 50% maximal stenosis. An occlusion of one calf artery (3 points) and more than 50% stenosis in another calf artery (2.5 points) already implies compromised runoff. Bad runoff with a score of 11 or more points after femoropopliteal PTA implies complete occlusion of all 3 calf arteries plus at least 20–49% residual stenosis of the popliteal artery. Some typical examples of infrapopliteal runoff scoring are shown in Figure 1.

All subjects have examined by vascular ultrasonography (US) at 1 month (range 29–60 days), 6 months (range 6–8 months), and 12 months (range 12–16 months) after PTA to evaluate the development of restenosis/reocclusion of the femoropoliteal arterial segment on a Vivid 3 ultrasound machine (GE Medical Systems, USA) with a linear vascular probe (Vascular 10L). An adverse outcome of PTA has defined as identification of femoropopliteal stenosis of ≥50%, confirmed by at least doubling of the maximal systolic velocity in comparison to a proximal nondiseased arterial segment, or by identifying a reocclusion confirmed by the absence of a Doppler flow signal [25]. The patency of calf arteries has been assessed by US at the third

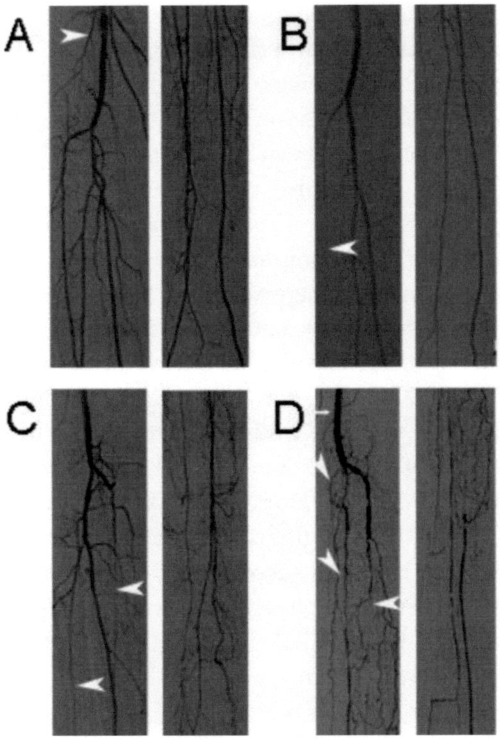

Figure 1. Examples of infrapopliteal scoring according to a modification of the Society for Vascular Surgery criteria [25]. In each set of angiograms, the left image represents the popliteal artery and the upper calf, while the right image represents the lower calf. (A) Good runoff with a score of 1: 3 × 0 + 1 point for a patent popliteal artery with <20% popliteal stenosis (arrowhead) plus 3 × 0 points for patent calf arteries. (B) Good runoff with a score of 4: 3 × 0 + 1 for the good patency of popliteal artery and 3 points for anterior tibial artery occlusion (arrowhead). (C) Compromised runoff with a score 5.5: 3 × 0 + 1 for good popliteal patency and 2 points for >50% posterior tibial artery stenosis (lower arrowhead) plus 2.5 points for anterior tibial artery occlusion spanning less than half of the arterial length (upper arrowhead). (D) Bad runoff with a score of 12: 3 × 1 + 1 points for 20–49% popliteal stenosis (small arrow) plus 2.5 points for occlusion of less than half of the length of the anterior tibial artery (lower horizontal arrowhead), plus 2.5 points for occlusion of less than half of the length of the peroneal artery with collateral filling (upper skewed arrowhead) plus 3 points for total occlusion of the posterior tibial artery with a collateral artery running along its path (lower skewed arrowhead). Reproduced with permission from [22].

follow-up examination 12 months after femoropopliteal PTA and compared to the periprocedural angiographic result. During US of the calf arteries, attempts have been made at visualizing as much as possible of the whole length of the two tibial arteries and the peroneal artery, i.e., interosseal artery. As in the femoropopliteal arterial segment, a stenosis of ≥50% has been diagnosed by at least doubling of the maximal systolic velocity in comparison to a proximal nondiseased arterial segment, whereas an occlusion has been documented in the absence of Doppler flow signal. In addition, the Doppler waveform at the level of the ankle in each of the three calf arteries has been compared to the waveform in the tibioperoneal trunk. A change from triphasic to monophasic signal with a marked reduction in peak systolic velocity and a decrease in the slope of systolic upstroke or absence of distal flow have been taken as additional evidence of hemodynamically significant compromise of the investigated calf artery [25].

Patients' blood has been collected 1 day before PTA (preprocedural sample) and on the day of PTA after the procedure (postprocedural sample). Blood has been drawn into 4.5 mL Vacutainer® tubes (Becton Dickinson, Plymouth, UK) containing 0.11 mol/L sodium citrate. From whole blood, DNA has been extracted either manually utilizing the silica-membrane-based DNA purification (QIAamp DNA Blood Mini Kit, Qiagen, Germany) or with magnetic beads on an automated nucleic acid purification instrument with the iPrep™ PureLink® gDNA Blood Kit (Life Technologies, USA). The remaining blood has been centrifuged at 2,000*g* and 4°C for 30 min to obtain platelet-poor plasma. Plasma has been transferred to small plastic vials, frozen in liquid nitrogen, and stored at –70°C until analyzed.

Genotyping of prothrombotic polymorphisms (GPIIIa T1565C, factor V G1691A, factor II G20210A, factor XII C46T and PAI-1 4G5G) and NuRR1 has been performed with real-time PCR on an ABI PRISM 7000 system (Applied Biosystems), using TaqMan® chemistry. In plasma, thrombin generation and D-dimer levels have been measured. Thrombin generation has been determined using a commercial kit (Technothrombin® TGA, Technoclone, Austria), which is based on monitoring the fluorescence generated by thrombin cleavage of a fluorogenic substrate over time on the activation of the coagulation cascade with 5 pmol/L tissue factor. The following parameters have been registered: lag phase, time to peak thrombin concentration, peak thrombin concentration and area under the curve–endogenous thrombin potential (ETP). The amount of microparticle-induced thrombin generation has also been determined by measuring thrombin generation in microparticle-free (filtered using 0.2 μm vacuum filtration device Ceveron® MFU-500, Technoclone, Austria) plasma versus thrombin generation in nonfiltered plasma containing microparticles. The amount of thrombin (peak thrombin concentration) induced by microparticles has been calculated (in per cent). D-dimer concentration has been measured with TriniLIA Auto-Dimer reagent (Trinity Biotech, Ireland) on an automated coagulation analyzer CS2100i (Siemens Healthcare Diagnostics, Germany) [27].

4. Results and discussion

4.1. Infrapopliteal runoff

Data on the infrapopliteal runoff have been analyzed for 176 patients [22]. We found a significantly higher restenosis/reocclusion rate in patients with compromised runoff (23%) compared to patients with a good runoff (11%) 1 month after femoropopliteal PTA ($p = 0.03$, Figure 2) [22]. The statistical significance was lost later on (after 6 months 49% in the compromised runoff group vs. 43% in the good runoff group, $p = 0.49$ and 57% vs. 52% after 12 months, respectively, $p = 0.51$). However, in patients' limbs with good periprocedural runoff that deteriorated into compromised runoff in the year after PTA, femoropopliteal restenosis/reocclusion occurred more often than in limbs which retained good runoff: 10/14 (71%) vs. 18/51 (35%), $p = 0.02$ [22]. The results were similar if only patients with Fontaine stages III and IV, i.e., critical limb ischemia were regarded. These results suggest that mechanisms of intermediate and long-term restenosis/reocclusion act simultaneously in the calf and the femoropopliteal arterial segment. The higher rate of early femoropopliteal restenosis/reocclusion after PTA in limbs with compromised infrapopliteal runoff could at least in part be the consequence of a diminished arterial blood flow predisposing to thrombosis. We recorded four early femoropopliteal reocclusions among limbs with compromised infrapopliteal runoff and one early reocclusion among patients' limbs with good runoff, but due to small number, the difference was not statistically significant. Our results at 6 and 12 months suggest that the postprocedural infrapopliteal runoff is not a prognostic indicator of intermediate and late restenosis/reocclusion, which are mainly caused by neointimal hyperplasia and advancing atherosclerosis.

In interpreting these results, we must keep in mind that 40% of the subjects had their infrapopliteal runoff improved by PTA, and that our study tested the effects of postprocedural not preprocedural runoff of diseased arterial segments [22]. In this respect, our work differs from previous studies that found poor runoff strongly predictive of a bad long-term outcome of femoropopliteal PTA [57] and agrees with the finding of no effect of tibial runoff on the rate of the 1-year patency of recanalized superficial femoral artery occlusions in patients with at least 1 patent tibial artery in the affected limb [11]. When we calculated the outcomes with respect to preprocedural runoff, we found no association between the rate of restenosis/reocclusion and the infrapopliteal runoff before it was improved by PTA [22]. This finding in combination with our results according to postprocedural runoff strongly suggests that improving the infrapopliteal runoff by PTA delays the time to femoropopliteal restenosis/reocclusion, which may be especially beneficial in cases of critical limb ischemia. Patients' limbs that experienced deterioration of good postprocedural infrapopliteal runoff in the first year after PTA were affected by an approximately doubled rate of restenosis/reocclusion of the femoropopliteal artery in comparison with limbs that retained good runoff [22]. This means that worsening of infrapopliteal runoff was accompanied not only by early but also by intermediate and late femoropopliteal restenosis or reocclusion, probably due to neointimal hyperplasia and progression of atherosclerotic disease.

The combined complication rate of the PTA in our patients was 7%: 3 minor heamatomas, 2 pseudoaneurysms (managed by conservative treatment), and 1 periprocedural thrombosis. The average ABI improved from 0.60 ± 0.41 before PTA to 0.82 ± 0.25 after PTA ($p < 0.001$). Among the 176 treated patients, 3 had minor limb amputations within 1 month after PTA (2 transmetatarsal and 1 toe amputation), 4 additional patients had limb amputations within 6 months (2 above the knee and 2 below the knee), and 5 additional patients within 12 months (2 above the knee, 2 below the knee, and 1 with an undisclosed level of amputation). Overall, the amputation rate was 12/176 patients (7%) after 1 year. Two patients died within 6 months after PTA and a total of 8/176 patients (5%) died within the first year [22]. Overall, our results with a combined femoropopliteal restenosis/reocclusion rate of 55% and a reocclusion rate of 21% 1 year after PTA [22] were comparable to the published data for patients without implantation of self-expanding femoral stents [24, 28].This was expected since we used femoral stents only for bailout indications, i.e., in 3 out of 176 treated patients' limbs. The clinical success of PTA among our series of patients was demonstrated by the low 1-year amputation rate despite the advanced stages of PAD among our patients (36% in Fontaine stage III with rest pain and 40% in Fontaine stage IV with skin ulcerations). This result is at the upper level of the reported limb salvage rate with traditional recanalization techniques [29].

Among our patients, no significant differences in postprocedural runoff were found with respect to the presence of diabetes or renal failure, but there were more smokers in the group with compromised postprocedural runoff in comparison to the group with good runoff and more patients with hypercholesterolemia [22]. While smoking might have decreased the feasibility of infrapopliteal PTA, the greater prevalence of hypercholesterolemia among patients with compromised postprocedural runoff could be just a chance finding, although hypercholesterolemia has been associated with restenosis of TASC B and C femoropopliteal lesions after PTA [30].

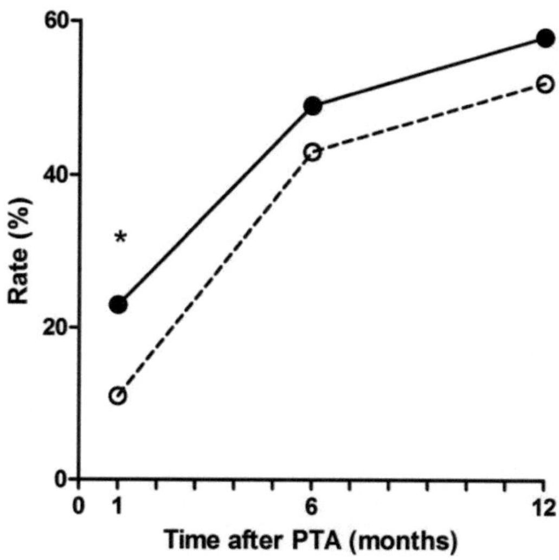

Figure 2. Time course of restenosis/reocclusion rates (%) in compromised runoff (full circle) and restenosis/reocclusion in good runoff (empty circle). Reproduced with permission from [22]. $^{*}p < 0.03$

4.2. Hemostasis

To detect a possible prothrombotic state in patients referred for femoropopliteal PTA, thrombin generation and D-dimer concentration were measured before and after PTA in 88 patients. Thrombin generation assay indicates the potential of plasma to generate thrombin following the in vitro activation of coagulation with tissue factor or another trigger. The resulting thrombin generation curve reflects all pro- and anticoagulant reactions that regulate the formation and inhibition of thrombin [31]. D-dimer is a specific degradation product of cross-linked fibrin and is thus a marker of both activated coagulation and fibrinolysis. D-dimer is best known today as the biochemical gold standard for initial assessment of hypercoagulability in suspected venous thrombosis [32].

We detected a hemostatic shift toward hypercoagulability induced by PTA by a significantly higher postprocedurel thrombin generation expressed by increased ETP and higher D-dimer concentration compared to preprocedural values (Table 1). However, we found association neither between thrombin generation nor D-dimer (either before or after PTA) and restenosis/reocclusion rate. No association between preprocedural thrombin generation and restenosis rate has also been observed in another study [33]. On the other hand, preprocedural hypercoagulability detected as shortening of the thromboelastometry-derived coagulation time (<444.5 s) reliably identified patients with high-degree in-stent restenosis in the superficial femoral artery [34]. Higher levels of preprocedural fibrinogen were also documented in patients with restenosis compared to patients with patent arteries [35].

	Before PTA	After PTA	p
Thrombin generation			
Lag phase (min)	10.8 ± 2.5	10.8 ± 2.2	NS
Peak thrombin (nM)	385 ± 96	393 ± 80	NS
Time to peak (min)	13.6 ± 3.1	13.8 ± 2.6	NS
Velocity	157 ± 83	154 ± 81	NS
ETP	3559 ± 542	3739 ± 490	<0.001
Microparticles (%)	26.8 ± 11.1	26.0 ± 10.2	NS
D-dimer (μg/L)	168 (99–479)	242 (138–584)	<0.001

ETP—endogenous thrombin potential, NS—not significant.

Table 1. Thrombin generation and D-dimer before and after PTA (mean ± standard deviation with Student's paired *t*-test *p* or median, 1st–3rd quartile with Wilcoxon signed-rank test *p*).

Genotyping of the prothrombotic polymorphisms was performed in 128 patients. All the tested polymorphisms were equally distributed among patients with or without restenosis/reocclusion in the first year after PTA (Table 2), suggesting that these polymorphisms have probably no major role in restenosis/reocclusion [36]. However, in order to detect possible weak association between these polymorphisms and femoropopliteal restenosis/reocclusion rate after PTA, a larger study population would be required.

With the exception of the study showing association of factor V G1691A with failed vascular reconstructions in patients with PTA [37], associations between prothrombotic gene polymorphisms and the risk of restenosis have been studied predominantly after percutaneous transluminal coronary angioplasty (PTCA). GPIIIa T1565C polymorphism was associated with higher risk of stent thrombosis after revascularization [38, 39] and with restenosis after PTCA in some [40], but not other studies [41]. Among other prothrombotic polymorphisms, factor V G1691A and PAI-1 4G5G may also play a role in the process of restenosis after PTCA. The PAI-1 4G variant was associated with an increased risk of restenosis after this procedure in contrast to factor V G1691A, which decreased the risk [42]. As far as we know, there has been no studies on the association of GPIIIa T1565C, factor II G20210A, factor XII C46T, and PAI-1 4G5G polymorphism with restenosis/reocclusion after PTA.

http://dx.doi.org/10.5772/61519

Polymorphism		Restenosis/reocclusion (N = 74)	Patent arteries (N = 54)	*p*
GP IIIa T1565C				
Genotype	TT	45 (61)	35 (65)	
	TC	27 (36)	17 (31)	NS
	CC	2 (3)	2 (4)	
1565C allele frequency		0.20	0.21	
FVL G1691A				
Genotype	GG	71 (96)	51 (94)	
	AG	3 (4)	3 (6)	NS
	AA	0 (0)	0 (0)	
1691A allele frequency		0.02	0.03	NS
Factor II G20210A				
Genotype	GG	70 (95)	53 (98)	
	AG	4 (5)	1 (2)	NS
	AA	0 (0)	0 (0)	
20210A allele frequency		0.01	0.03	NS
PAI-1 4G5G				
Genotype	5G5G	21 (28)	6 (11)	
	4G5G	22 (30)	29 (54)	NS
	4G4G	31 (42)	19 (35)	
4G allele frequency		0.62	0.57	
FXII C46T				
Genotype	CC	46 (62)	33 (61)	
	CT	23 (31)	18 (33)	NS
	TT	5 (7)	3 (6)	
FXII 46T allele frequency		0.77	0.72	NS

NS—not significant.

Table 2. Genotype in allele distribution in patients with restenosis/reocclusion or patients with patent arteries in the first year after PTA.

4.3. Inflammation

Genotyping of the three tagging single-nucleotide polymorphisms (rs1466408, rs13428968, and rs12803) in the NuRR1 gene was performed in 142 patients with femoropopliteal PTA who finished a 12-month follow-up. From these three polymorphisms, four haplotypes were inferred as described earlier, and their frequencies were similar to that earlier observed in Caucasian population [20]. Haplotype 1 was the most frequent and served as the reference haplotype. Haplotypes 2 and 3 significantly increased the restenosis/reocclusion rate as shown by the relative risks adjusted for sex, age, and Fontaine classification calculated by Cox regression (Table 3) [43].

Haplotype	rs1466408	rs13428968	rs12803	Frequency (%)	Relative risk (95% CI)
Haplotype 1	T	T	G	49.4	-
Haplotype 2	T	T	T	23.3	1.6 (1.1–2.3)
Haplotype 3	T	C	T	19.7	2.0 (1.3–2.8)
Haplotype 4	A	T	T	6.6	NS

CI—confidence interval, NS—not significant.

Table 3. Composition and frequencies of the 4 NuRR1 haplotypes with frequencies >1% and adjusted relative risk associated with each haplotype in our study population.

Similar to our study, haplotype 3 increased the risk of in-stent restenosis, target lesion revascularization, percutaneous coronary interventions, and the rate of MACE about 2-fold in the first year after the procedure [20]. This study reported no association of haplotype 2, while haplotype 4 increased the risk of in-stent restenosis, target lesion revascularization, percutaneous coronary interventions, and the rate of MACE about 2- to 3-fold in the first year after the procedure [20]. We were not able to confirm an increased risk of restenosis/reocclusion in patients with haplotype 4 probably due to the small number of patients with this haplotype, and further analysis on a larger group of patients is warranted.

Despite a well-recognized role of inflammation in restenosis and known polymorphisms in inflammation marker genes that influence their level or function, the influence of these polymorphisms on restenosis rate has not yet been extensively studied. In addition, most studies to date focused on patients with PTCA rather than PTA. Among the most extensively studied polymorphisms is the angiotensin-converting enzyme (ACE) insertion/deletion (I/D) polymorphism in intron 16 of the ACE gene. Meta-analysis of 33 cohort studies involving 11,099 subjects confirmed that carriers of the ACE DD genotype are subjected to a significantly increased risk (odds ratio 1.61, 95% CI 1.27–2.04, $p < 0.001$) for post-PTCA restenosis [44].

In patients with femoropopliteal PTA, two studies were reported that involved gene polymorphisms in interleukins. In the first study, a combined effect of the interleukin-1B C(-511)T single-nucleotide polymorphism and a variable number tandem repeat polymorphism in intron 2 of the interleukin-1 receptor antagonist gene (IL-1RN VNTR) were associated with a higher restenosis risk [45]. In the second study, a 2.4-fold increased adjusted risk for restenosis was observed in carriers of the interleukin-6 (-174)CC genotype compared to carriers of the (-174)GG genotype [46].

5. Conclusion

Our understanding of the mechanisms of restenosis/reocclusion of the femoral artery after PTA is deficient, and this study provided some additional evidence on the subject. The study suggested a significantly higher restenosis/reocclusion rate in patients with compromised runoff compared to patients with a good runoff 1 month after the procedure. In all patients, hypercoagulability as assessed by a thrombin generation assay and D-dimer was observed after PTA but was not associated with the restenosis/reocclusion rate. Prothrombotic polymorphisms were equally distributed among patient with and without restenosis/reocclusion suggesting minor or no role of these polymorphisms in the risk of restenosis/reocclusion. On the other hand, haplotypes 2 and 3 in the NuRR1 gene significantly increased the restenosis/reocclusion rate, suggesting significant role of inflammation. In this ongoing study, further analysis on a larger group of patients is warranted, and possible consideration of combinations of genetic markers rather than isolated polymorphisms in the analysis of this multifactorial vascular disease might provide further evidence on the risk of restenosis/reocclusion after PTA.

Acknowledgements

The study is supported by the Slovenian Research Agency (grant no. P3-0308).

Author details

Mojca Božič-Mijovski[1*], Vinko Boc[1], Vladka Salapura[2], Aleš Blinc[1,2] and Mojca Stegnar[1]

*Address all correspondence to: mojca.bozic@kclj.si

1 Department of Vascular Diseases, University Medical Centre Ljubljana, Ljubljana, Slovenia

2 Institute of Radiology, University Medical Centre Ljubljana and Faculty of Medicine, University of Ljubljana, Ljubljana, Slovenia

References

[1] Criqui MH, Langer RD, Fronek A, Feigelson HS, Klauber MR, McCann TJ, Browner D. Mortality over a period of 10 years in patients with peripheral arterial disease. New England Journal of Medicine 1992;326: 381–6.

[2] Hirsch AT, Criqui MH, Treat-Jacobson D, Regensteiner JG, Creager MA, Olin JW, Krook SH, Hunninghake DB, Comerota AJ, Walsh ME, McDermott MM, Hiatt WR.

Peripheral arterial disease detection, awareness, and treatment in primary care. JAMA 2001;286: 1317–24.

[3] European Stroke O, Tendera M, Aboyans V, Bartelink ML, Baumgartner I, Clement D, Collet JP, Cremonesi A, De Carlo M, Erbel R, Fowkes FG, Heras M, Kownator S, Minar E, Ostergren J, Poldermans D, Riambau V, Roffi M, Rother J, Sievert H, van Sambeek M, Zeller T, Guidelines ESCCfP. ESC guidelines on the diagnosis and treatment of peripheral artery diseases: document covering atherosclerotic disease of extracranial carotid and vertebral, mesenteric, renal, upper and lower extremity arteries: the Task Force on the Diagnosis and Treatment of Peripheral Artery Diseases of the European Society of Cardiology (ESC). European Heart Journal 2011;32: 2851–906.

[4] Norgren L, Hiatt WR, Dormandy JA, Nehler MR, Harris KA, Fowkes FG, Group TIW. Inter-society consensus for the management of peripheral arterial disease (TASC II). Journal of Vascular Surgery 2007;45(Suppl S): S5–67.

[5] Matsi PJ, Manninen HI, Vanninen RL, Suhonen MT, Oksala I, Laakso M, Hakkarainen T, Soimakallio S. Femoropopliteal angioplasty in patients with claudication: primary and secondary patency in 140 limbs with 1–3-year follow-up. Radiology 1994;191: 727–33.

[6] Clark TW, Groffsky JL, Soulen MC. Predictors of long-term patency after femoropopliteal angioplasty: results from the STAR registry. Journal of Vascular Interventional Radiology 2001;12: 923–33.

[7] Johnston KW. Femoral and popliteal arteries: reanalysis of results of balloon angioplasty. Radiology 1992;183: 767–71.

[8] Krepel VM, van Andel GJ, van Erp WF, Breslau PJ. Percutaneous transluminal angioplasty of the femoropopliteal artery: initial and long-term results. Radiology 1985;156: 325–8.

[9] Matsi PJ, Manninen HI, Suhonen MT, Pirinen AE, Soimakallio S. Chronic critical lower-limb ischemia: prospective trial of angioplasty with 1–36 months follow-up. Radiology 1993;188: 381–7.

[10] Stokes KR, Strunk HM, Campbell DR, Gibbons GW, Wheeler HG, Clouse ME. Five-year results of iliac and femoropopliteal angioplasty in diabetic patients. Radiology 1990;174: 977–82.

[11] Gordon IL, Conroy RM, Tobis JM, Kohl C, Wilson SE. Determinants of patency after percutaneous angioplasty and atherectomy of occluded superficial femoral arteries. American Journal of Surgery 1994;168: 115–9.

[12] Fuster V, Falk E, Fallon JT, Badimon L, Chesebro JH, Badimon JJ. The three processes leading to Post PTCA restenosis: dependence on the lesion substrate. Thrombosis and Haemostasis 1995;74: 552–9.

[13] Ten Cate H. Thrombin generation in clinical conditions. Thrombosis Research 2012;129: 367–70.

[14] Vižintin Cuderman T, Božič M, Peternel P, Stegnar M. Hemostasis activation in thrombophilic subjects with or without a history of venous thrombosis. Clinical and Applied Thrombosis and Hemostasis 2008;14: 55–62.

[15] Chistiakov DA, Orekhov AN, Bobryshev YV. Vascular smooth muscle cell in atherosclerosis. Acta Physiologica (Oxf) 2015.

[16] Schillinger M, Minar E. Restenosis after percutaneous angioplasty: the role of vascular inflammation. Vascular Health Risk Management 2005;1: 73–8.

[17] Mickelson JK, Lakkis NM, Villarreal-Levy G, Hughes BJ, Smith CW. Leukocyte activation with platelet adhesion after coronary angioplasty: a mechanism for recurrent disease? Journal of the American College of Cardiology 1996;28: 345–53.

[18] Bonta PI, Pols TW, de Vries CJ. Nr4a nuclear receptors in atherosclerosis and vein-graft disease. Trends in Cardiovascular Medicine 2007;17: 105–11.

[19] Bonta PI, van Tiel CM, Vos M, Pols TW, van Thienen JV, Ferreira V, Arkenbout EK, Seppen J, Spek CA, van der Poll T, Pannekoek H, de Vries CJ. Nuclear receptors Nur77, Nurr1, and nor-1 expressed in atherosclerotic lesion macrophages reduce lipid loading and inflammatory responses. Arteriosclerosis, Thrombosis, and Vascular Biology 2006;26: 2288–94.

[20] Bonta PI, Pols TW, van Tiel CM, Vos M, Arkenbout EK, Rohlena J, Koch KT, de Maat MP, Tanck MW, de Winter RJ, Pannekoek H, Biessen EA, Bot I, de Vries CJ. Nuclear receptor Nurr1 is expressed in and is associated with human restenosis and inhibits vascular lesion formation in mice involving inhibition of smooth muscle cell proliferation and inflammation. Circulation 2010;121: 2023–32.

[21] Kardys I, van Tiel CM, de Vries CJ, Pannekoek H, Uitterlinden AG, Hofman A, Witteman JC, de Maat MP. Haplotypes of the Nr4a2/Nurr1 gene and cardiovascular disease: the Rotterdam Study. Human Mutation 2009;30: 417–23.

[22] Salapura V, Blinc A, Kozak M, Ježovnik MK, Pohar Perme M, Berden P, Kuhelj D, Ključevšek T, Popovič P, Stankovič M, Vrtovec M, Šurlan M. Infrapopliteal run-off and the outcome of femoropopliteal percutaneous transluminal angioplasty. Vasa 2010;39: 159–68.

[23] Orchard TJ, Strandness DE, Jr. Assessment of peripheral vascular disease in diabetes. Report and recommendations of an international workshop sponsored by the American Diabetes Association and the American Heart Association September 18–20, 1992 New Orleans, Louisiana. Circulation 1993;88: 819–28.

[24] Schillinger M, Sabeti S, Loewe C, Dick P, Amighi J, Mlekusch W, Schlager O, Cejna M, Lammer J, Minar E. Balloon angioplasty versus implantation of nitinol stents in the superficial femoral artery. New England Journal of Medicine 2006;354: 1879–88.

[25] MacAllister, L. Peripheral Vascular Sonography. Philadelphia: Lippincott Williams and Wilkins; 2004.

[26] Rutherford RB, Baker JD, Ernst C, Johnston KW, Porter JM, Ahn S, Jones DN. Recommended standards for reports dealing with lower extremity ischemia: revised version. Journal of Vascular Surgery 1997;26: 517–38.

[27] Božič M, Stegnar M. Validation of an automated immunoturbidimetric assay for measurement of plasma D-dimer. Clinical Chemistry and Laboratory Medicine 2003;41: 958–62.

[28] Schillinger M, Minar E. Endovascular stent implantation for treatment of peripheral artery disease. European Journal of Clinical Investigation 2007;37: 165–70.

[29] Zeller T, Sixt S, Rastan A. New techniques for endovascular treatment of peripheral artery disease with focus on chronic critical limb ischemia. Vasa 2009;38: 3–12.

[30] Baril DT, Marone LK, Kim J, Go MR, Chaer RA, Rhee RY. Outcomes of endovascular interventions for TASC II B and C femoropopliteal lesions. Journal of Vascular Surgery 2008;48: 627–33.

[31] Hemker HC, Giesen P, AlDieri R, Regnault V, de Smed E, Wagenvoord R, Lecompte T, Beguin S. The calibrated automated thrombogram (CAT): a universal routine test for hyper- and hypocoagulability. Pathophysiology of Haemostasis and Thrombosis 2002;32: 249–53.

[32] Righini M, Perrier A, De Moerloose P, Bounameaux H. D-Dimer for venous thromboembolism diagnosis: 20 years later. Journal of Thrombosis and Haemostasis 2008;6: 1059–71.

[33] Gremmel T, Koppensteiner R, Ay C, Panzer S. Residual thrombin generation potential is inversely linked to the occurrence of atherothrombotic events in patients with peripheral arterial disease. European Journal of Clinical Investigation 2014;44: 319–324.

[34] Cvirn G, Hoerl G, Schlagenhauf A, Tafeit E, Brodmann M, Juergens G, Koestenberger M, Gary T. Stent implantation in the superficial femoral artery: short thrombelastometry-derived coagulation times identify patients with late in-stent restenosis. Thrombosis Research 2012;130: 485–90.

[35] Tschopl M, Tsakiris DA, Marbet GA, Labs KH, Jager K. Role of hemostatic risk factors for restenosis in peripheral arterial occlusive disease after transluminal angioplasty. Arteriosclerosis, Thrombosis, and Vascular Biology 1997;17: 3208–14.

[36] Bedenčič M, Božič M, Salapura V, Blinc A, Stegnar M. Genetic predisposition to the risk of restenosis after femoropopliteal percutaneous transluminal angioplasty. Pathophysiology of Haemostasis and Thrombosis 2008;36:A41.

[37] Sampram ES, Lindblad B, Dahlback B. Activated protein C resistance in patients with peripheral vascular disease. Journal of Vascular Surgery 1998;28: 624–9.

[38] Di Castelnuovo A, de Gaetano G, Donati MB, Iacoviello L. Platelet glycoprotein receptor IIIA polymorphism Pla1/Pla2 and coronary risk: a meta-analysis. Thrombosis and Haemostasis 2001;85: 626–33.

[39] Williams MS, Bray PF. Genetics of arterial prothrombotic risk states. Experimental Biology and Medicine (Maywood) 2001;226: 409–19.

[40] Abbate R, Marcucci R, Camacho-Vanegas O, Pepe G, Gori AM, Capanni M, Simonetti I, Prisco D, Gensini GF. Role of platelet glycoprotein Pl(A1/A2) polymorphism in restenosis after percutaneous transluminal coronary angioplasty. American Journal of Cardiology 1998;82: 524–5.

[41] Mamotte CD, van Bockxmeer FM, Taylor RR. Pia1/A2 polymorphism of glycoprotein IIIA and risk of coronary artery disease and restenosis following coronary angioplasty. American Journal of Cardiology 1998;82: 13–6.

[42] Pons D, Monraats PS, de Maat MP, Pires NM, Quax PH, van Vlijmen BJ, Rosendaal FR, Zwinderman AH, Doevendans PA, Waltenberger J, de Winter RJ, Tio RA, Frants RR, van der Laarse A, van der Wall EE, Jukema JW. The influence of established genetic variation in the haemostatic system on clinical restenosis after percutaneous coronary interventions. Thrombosis and Haemostasis 2007;98: 1323–8.

[43] Božič-Mijovski M, Bedenčič M, Stegnar M, Salapura V, Ježovnik MK, Kozak M, Blinc A. Nurr1 haplotypes are associated with femoropopliteal restenosis/re-occlusion after percutaneous transluminal angioplasty. European Journal of Vascular and Endovascular Surgery 2012;43: 337–8.

[44] Wang S, Dai Y, Chen L, Dong Z, Chen Y, Li C, Zhong X, Lin W, Zhang J. Genetic polymorphism of angiotensin converting enzyme and risk of coronary restenosis after percutaneous transluminal coronary angioplasties: evidence from 33 cohort studies. PloS One 2013;8: e75285.

[45] Marculescu R, Mlekusch W, Exner M, Sabeti S, Michor S, Rumpold H, Mannhalter C, Minar E, Wagner O, Schillinger M. Interleukin-1 cluster combined genotype and restenosis after balloon angioplasty. Thrombosis and Haemostasis 2003;90: 491–500.

[46] Exner M, Schillinger M, Minar E, Mlekusch W, Sabeti S, Endler G, Raith M, Mannhalter C, Wagner O. Interleukin-6 promoter genotype and restenosis after femoropopliteal balloon angioplasty: initial observations. Radiology 2004;231: 839–44.

Chapter 5

Common Gene Polymorphisms Associated with Thrombophilia

Christos Yapijakis, Zoe Serefoglou and Constantinos Voumvourakis

Additional information is available at the end of the chapter

http://dx.doi.org/10.5772/61859

Abstract

Genetic association studies have revealed a correlation between DNA variations in genes encoding factors of the hemostatic system and thrombosis-related disease. Certain variant alleles of these genes that affect either gene expression or function of encoded protein are known to be genetic risk factors for thrombophilia. The chapter presents the current genetics and molecular biology knowledge of the most important DNA polymorphisms in thrombosis-related genes encoding coagulation factor V (FV), coagulation factor II (FII), coagulation factor XII (FXII), coagulation factor XIII A1 subunit (FXIIIA1), 5,10-methylene tetrahydrofolate reductase (MTHFR), serpine1 (SERPINE1), angiotensin I-converting enzyme (ACE), angiotensinogen (AGT), integrin A2 (ITGA2), plasma carboxypeptidase B2 (CPB2), platelet glycoprotein Ib α polypeptide (GP1BA), thrombomodulin (THBD) and protein Z (PROZ). The molecular detection methods of each DNA polymorphism is presented, in addition to the current knowledge regarding its influence on thrombophilia and related thrombotic events, including stroke, myocardial infarction, deep vein thrombosis, spontaneous abortion, etc. In addition, best thrombosis prevention strategies with a combination of genetic counseling and molecular testing are discussed.

Keywords: Thrombophilia, coagulation factors, genetic association, DNA polymorphisms, molecular analysis

1. Introduction

Thrombosis is a common underlying pathological event of venous thromboembolism, ischemic stroke and ischemic heart disorder. It is well established that all three diseases are associated with a major global burden [1, 2]. Thrombophilia (a Greek composite word including "thrombos" meaning clot and "philia" meaning friendship) is a condition where individual susceptibility to thrombotic disease due to deregulation of the hemostatic system is known to be influenced by several hereditary and lifestyle-related factors [3–5]. Genetic association studies have revealed a correlation between DNA variations in genes encoding factors of the hemostatic system and thrombosis-related disease [6–10].

Certain variant alleles of these thrombosis-associated genes that affect either gene expression or function of encoded protein are known to be genetic risk factors for thrombophilia. The genetic variants are found in genes involved in coagulation, fibrinolysis, platelet activity and other functions related to thrombosis [4, 9, 11]. Most of these are single-nucleotide polymorphisms (SNPs) and affect hemostatic mechanisms in a quantitative or in a qualitative manner [9, 11]. Primary and secondary prevention of death and disability incidence due to thrombotic events may be effected through optimized anticoagulant treatment at individual patient level. This chapter will discuss the current molecular biology and genetics knowledge of the most important DNA polymorphisms in thrombosis-related genes. In addition, best thrombosis prevention strategies with a combination of genetic counseling and molecular testing will be discussed.

2. Coagulation and thrombosis-related factors

Coagulation is a complex multienzymatic cascade by which fibrin is produced forming the basis of a clot. Thrombosis involves an imbalance of coagulation and fibrinolysis, which also includes formation and degradation of extracellular matrix (ECM).

The most essential components of the coagulation and fibrinolysis systems are associated with the endothelial cell membrane, including tissue factor (TF), thrombin and urokinase receptors. They become exposed when vessels are injured and when platelets are bound to them at early stages of either coagulation or inflammation. Consequently, platelets release vascular endothelial growth factor (VEGF) and other growth factors into the circulation, thus promoting angiogenesis and attracting inflammatory cells to the site of injury [12]. In addition, platelets also contain hemostatic factors that regulate the extent of tissue repair and inhibit vascularization, such as serpine1, previously known as plasminogen activator inhibitor-1 (PAI-1) [12].

The coagulatory cascade is artificially divided based on *in vitro* testing in the intrinsic or contact pathway and the extrinsic or tissue factor (TF) pathway. The two pathways interfere since both thrombin and TF may activate coagulation factor IX (FIX) [12].

3. Tissue factor pathway

TF is expressed constitutively on subendothelial fibroblasts and smooth muscle cells which are exposed to blood only upon vascular damage. Therefore, TF acts as the physiological initiator of coagulation [13]. In addition, TF is expressed on peripheral blood monocytes and on vascular endothelia after exposure to inflammatory or activating stimuli, such as endotoxin.

TF is a transmembrane glycoprotein with an extracellular ligand-binding domain that interacts with coagulation factor VII in both its inactive and active forms (FVII/FVIIa) [14]. When TF-expressing cells in extravascular sites come in contact with plasma, a complex of TF with the circulating FVII is formed on the cell surface, which is further activated to FVIIa by limited proteolysis, producing activated coagulation factor X (FXa) and thrombin and leading to coagulation. The function of TF is kept at appropriate levels through TF pathway inhibitor (TFPI), a protease inhibitor constitutively released from endothelia. TFPI interacts with circulating FXa and the TFPI/FXa complex binds to the TF/FVIIa complex down-regulating TF-induced quaternary complex of Ca^{2+} and coagulation factors VIIIa, IXa and X [15].

In addition to its hemostatic role, TF is also involved in normal embryonic angiogenesis through the induction of vascular endothelial growth factor (VEGF) and the secretion up-regulation of urokinase plasminogen activator receptor [16–18]. Both TF and VEGF are stimulated by hypoxia through different pathways [19, 20].

4. Thrombin pathway

Thrombin plays a central role in coagulation, since it is the most effective agonist for platelet activation and leads to the formation of the fibrin clot by activating various zymogens and cofactors, including fibrinogen, coagulation factors XIII, V and VIII, platelet membrane GPV, protein S and protein C [21]. Much like TF, thrombin may promote angiogenesis through different pathways and independently of fibrin generation.

Thrombin also enhances the migratory potential of endothelia through basement membranes by activating gelatinase A (matrix metalloprotenase-2, MMP-2), which degrades collagen IV and releases tissue plasminogen (t-PA) and PAI-1 [22–25]. In addition, thrombin activates platelets, leading to their aggregation and release of numerous pro- and anti-angiogenic factors. Furthermore, angiogenesis is inhibited by the prothrombin kringle 2 domain as well as two prothrombin fragments (F1 and F2) generated during activation of thrombin [26, 27].

Thrombin inhibits dissolution of clots and modulates fibrinolysis through activation of thrombin activatable fibrinolysis inhibitor (TAFI). TAFI cleaves certain C-terminal lysine residues from fibrin, thereby preventing plasminogen, plasmin and t-PA from binding to fibrin [28].

Thrombin forms a complex with thrombomodulin, an endothelial cell membrane protein, leading to the activation of protein C. Consequently, activated protein C cleaves non-platelet-associated activated coagulation factors V and VII (FVa and FVIIa), thus down-regulating thrombin formation by inactivating the prothrombinase complex as well as the quaternary complex of Ca^{2+} and coagulation factors VIIIa, IXa and X. In addition to its anticoagulant role, thrombomodulin reduces fibrinolysis by activating TAFI in plasma [29]).

5. Fibrinogen, cross-linked fibrin and fibrinolysis

Fibrinogen plays a critical role in hemostasis. Following activation by thrombin, fibrinogen is subsequently cleaved to monomers of fibrin that are rapidly combined to form a fibrin matrix.

In addition, thrombin activates coagulation factor XIII (FXIII) that converts soluble fibrin into an insoluble polymer of fibrin. Activated FXIII also prevents fibrinolysis by linking α2-plasmin inhibitor to fibrin [30].

The fibrin gel promotes angiogenesis and cell growth, by providing a provisional matrix, enriched in growth factors which are protected from degradation, such as VEGF and insulin-like growth factor-1 [31, 32]. Furthermore, the fibrin gel provides a surface suitable for the prothrombinase assembly, a function platelets perform in intravascular clotting.

The provisional fibrin matrix undergoes remodeling and is transformed into mature connective tissue stroma, which in its constituent elements resembles the stroma of healing wounds [33, 34]. There is a balance between deposition of fibrin gel from clotting activation and its dissolution through activation of fibrinolysis [34]. Fibrinolytic activity depends on the balance between several factors including coagulation XIIa (FXIIa), which converts plasminogen to plasmin, plasminogen activators (PA) and their inhibitors, such as PAI-1 and α2-antiplasmin.

6. Angiogenesis

Angiogenesis (vascularization) involves a sequence of key events which include focal detachment of endothelial cells from the basement membrane, localized proteolytic degradation of the basement membrane and ECM invasion, leading to capillary tube formation and vascular remodeling [35]. Hemostatic mechanisms may influence angiogenesis directly or indirectly through a number of different pathways, involving the release of pro-angiogenic and anti-angiogenic factors from activated platelets. These angiogenesis-related factors, such as tumor necrosis factor-alpha (TNF-α), promote both formation of fibrin-rich ECM and thrombin signaling through activation of G-protein-coupled protease-activated receptors on the endothelial cell surface [21, 36].

7. Thrombosis and cancer

Cancer-related thrombosis represents a complex imbalance of coagulation and fibrinolysis, also involving the formation and degradation of ECM through interaction of angiogenesis-related factors [37–40]. Within a tumor, new vessels leak fibrin into the extravascular space and therefore persistently activate the coagulatory system, both locally and systemically, producing the clinical appearance of an unhealed wound [12, 41].

The disruption of hemostatic mechanisms is not merely a secondary effect of cancer but it appears to be a frequent event [41–43]. Sometimes, the activation of coagulation, such as venous thromboembolism, may even precede the clinical manifestations of cancer [42, 43]. It is well established that bleeding diathesis and systemic activation of the coagulation cascade contribute significantly to morbidity and mortality of patients with malignancies [44, 45].

8. Genetic association studies

Susceptibility in thrombophilia, like in all multifactorial diseases, implicates the interaction between environmental factors, such as diet or smoking, as well as genetic factors [46]. In the last couple of decades, population-based genetic association studies have been extensively investigating DNA polymorphisms in genes putatively involved in multifactorial diseases [39, 40, 46]. Such studies estimate the risk of developing a certain disease by comparing the frequency of polymorphic genotypes and allele frequencies between patients and matched healthy controls of the same population. A variant allele or a genotype is associated with increased risk for a disease when its detected frequency is significantly higher in cases than controls [47]. A significant association result indicates that the studied DNA polymorphism tested either directly affects the risk of a certain disease or acts as a genetic marker for a linked genetic variant that influences risk for that disease [47].

Genetic association studies usually investigate common SNPs in genes of cohorts of individuals. Over 10 million known SNPs are included in public databases and more of them are constantly identified. The frequency of the less common variant allele of SNPs in the general population is at least 1%, while mutations are usually much rarer. Therefore, due to their high incidence in the population, SNPs are usually very informative [39, 40, 46]. However, genetic association studies have to be conducted based on certain basic criteria, such as the adequate number of studied individuals, the gender ratio, age and ethnic compatibility of patients and healthy controls in order to avoid false positive and false negative results [46, 48]. The observed genotypic frequencies are considered representative of the population either of patients or healthy people if they are compatible with the Hardy–Weinberg equilibrium [49]. Highly significant associations replicated by a number of studies may be a useful tool for the prognosis and prevention of disease [40, 50].

The spectrum of coagulation and fibrinolysis factors and their respective encoding genes suggests that a great number of functional DNA polymorphisms might confer a major or minor risk of thrombosis [4, 7–11, 51, 52]. The most important DNA polymorphisms in thrombosis-related genes will be discussed, including those encoding (a) coagulation factors, (b) thrombin-related factors, (c) fibrinolysis-related factors, (d) platelet-adhesion factors and (e) other factors. A handful of variants in genes encoding for certain factors of the hemostatic system are positively known to confer a highly significant thrombotic phenotype, such as coagulation factor V (FV) Leiden, while for other variants there is only some emerging evidence implicating them in thrombotic disease, such as *serpine1* (*PAI-1*) 4G/5G.

Some of the thrombosis-associated variants are very common in different populations, such as *serpine1* (*PAI-1*) 4G/5G, which ranges between 42% and 54% worldwide [11]. Other polymorphic variants differ widely among populations, such as *thrombomodulin* (*THBD*) -G13A, which is extremely rare in Caucasians (<1%) and ranges between 8% and 19% in East Asians [53–59].

9. Coagulation factors

FV Leiden is probably the most important hereditary thrombosis-associated factor in Caucasians, with heterozygotes exhibiting up to 10-fold greater relative risk and Leiden homozygotes 50–100-fold greater relative risk of venous thrombosis [60, 61]. *FV* Leiden is responsible for 20–25% of isolated thrombotic events and for 40–45% of cases of familial thrombophilia and fetal loss [3, 62–64]. The *FV* gene encodes a plasma glycoprotein which is activated by thrombin/coagulation factor Xa (FXa) and subsequently converted into factor Va (FVa). The Leiden variant (mutation G1691A) destroys a cleavage site of the anticoagulant-activated protein C in FVa. This variant has a wide allelic frequency range (1–9%) in European populations, while it is virtually absent from non-Caucasian populations [11, 60, 65]. *FV* Leiden is thought to have arisen approximately 21,000 to 34,000 years ago in Caucasians [60].

The gene encoding coagulation factor II (*FII*) or prothrombin contains another common defect in its 3′ untranslated region (G20210A). FII is a plasma glycoprotein which is activated to thrombin by coagulation factors FXa and FVa. The G20210A mutation is related to elevated plasma prothrombin levels, and heterozygotes have up to fourfold increased risk of venous thrombosis [66, 67]. The variant allele has a frequency of 1.3–4.5% in Caucasian populations [11, 65–67].

A common DNA polymorphism in the gene encoding coagulation factor XII (*F12*) is C46T. The prevalence of the thrombosis-related 46T allele ranges between 18% and 37% in various populations [11, 68]. In the gene *F13A1* coding for coagulation factor XIII A1 subunit, a SNP results in amino acid substitution Val34Leu [69]. There is emerging evidence that the *F13* 34Leu allele confers protection against thrombosis [69]. The prevalence of this particular allele varies considerably between populations ranging between 13% and 28% [11, 69].

9.1. Thrombin-related factors

The prevalence of the thrombin-related SNPs thrombomodulin (*THBD*) -G13A and protein Z (*PROZ*)-A33G is low in Caucasian populations (<1% and 6%, respectively) [11, 54, 70]. Both SNPs are located in the promoter region of the respective genes and the variant alleles result in lower levels of gene expression and lower protein production of thrombomodulin and protein Z. The role of both DNA polymorphisms in susceptibility for thrombosis appears to be minor.

9.2. Fibrinolysis-related factors

Variants in genes of fibrinolysis-related factors such as serpine1 (also known as plasminogen activator inhibitor-1, PAI-1) and thrombin-activatable fibrinolysis inhibitor (TAFI, also known as plasma carboxypeptidase B2, CPB2) have been shown to have an association with increased risk of venous thrombosis and myocardial infarction to a diverse extent [56, 71, 72].

A deletion/insertion polymorphism (4G/5G) in the promoter of the *serpine1* gene interferes with regulation of its transcription [72]. The 4G allele binds only an activator, while the 5G allele binds both a repressor and an activator. Therefore, the presence of the 4G variant results in higher gene expression, increased inhibition of the plasminogen activators and decreased plasminogen conversion to plasmin. Several studies have indicated that 4G/4G homozygosity is a risk factor for deep vein thrombosis, myocardial infarction and miscarriage during pregnancy [71, 72]. The prevalence of 4G variant in various populations ranges from 31% to 63% [11, 71, 72].

The effect of the C1040T polymorphism on TAFI (CPB2) function and its modest role in thrombosis is well established [56, 73]. The C to T substitution at codon 325 leads to a Thr to Ile change, which has an impact on the thermal stability of the enzyme, resulting in longer half-life and increased overall antifibrinolytic activity [74]. The prevalence of the 1040T variant in Caucasians and East Asians (31–40%) is much higher than African populations (11%) [11].

9.3. Platelet-adhesion factors

The role of DNA polymorphisms in genes encoding for platelet-adhesion factors, regarding the risk for certain thrombotic diseases, remains still uncertain although a minor contribution may not yet be ruled out. Among the most promising polymorphisms, possibly associated with risk for cerebrovascular diseases, appear to be C807T in the *ITGA2* gene which encodes integrin A2, also known as platelet glycoprotein Ia and variable number of tandem repeats (VNTR) in the *GP1BA* gene which encodes platelet glycoprotein Ibα polypeptide [11, 53, 75].

9.4. Other factors

Methylenetetrahydrofolate reductase (MTHFR) is an enzyme that plays an important role in folate metabolism [76]. A C677T mutation in the *MTHFR* gene involves an alanine/valine change that renders the protein temperature sensitive and diminishes its activity, resulting in the pro-thrombotic condition of hyperhomocysteinemia, particularly when dietary intake of folate is inadequate [8, 77–79]. Homozygotes for the 677T allele account for 8.5% of the general population in Caucasians, and they are known to have a higher risk for thrombotic events [11, 80].

Two other factors that are related directly to blood pressure and indirectly to thrombotic events are angiotensinogen (AGT) and angiotensin-converting enzyme (ACE), two major players in the rennin–angiotensin system, a circulatory cascade primarily involved in the regulation of blood pressure and serum electrolytes. AGT is hydrolyzed into angiotensin I by rennin, which is subsequently converted to potent vasoconstrictor angiotensin II by ACE [81].

Among several DNA polymorphisms in the *AGT* gene, the only well-studied one is a SNP at codon 235 because it influences gene expression and therefore has been associated with hypertension and thrombosis [82–85]. It involves an amino acid substitution (methionine to threonine, M235T). The high gene expression T allele has been associated with increased hypertension and risk for thrombosis [11, 82–84, 86]. The prevalence of the T variant is higher in Africans and Asians (78%), while it is lower in Caucasians ranging between 34% and 55% [11, 86].

ACE activity is mainly determined by the insertion/deletion (I/D) polymorphism of a 287 bp Alu repeat sequence inside intron 16 of the *ACE* gene [87]. Homozygotes for the I allele may display as low as half of the plasma ACE level compared to the homozygotes for the D allele, whereas the ID heterozygotes display an intermediate level [88]. The presence of the D allele causes elevation in angiotensin II levels and results in higher blood pressure. The D allele frequency is more abundant in Europeans (49–58%) than Asians (32–34%) [11].

10. Molecular detection methodology

Molecular analysis of DNA polymorphisms is usually performed in samples of genomic DNA extracted from blood, saliva, tissue, hair, semen or any other biological material. DNA testing of blood or saliva samples is a common practice. As in all occasions of genetic testing, a signed informed consent has to be obtained from any individual whose DNA would be examined.

The molecular detection methods of each DNA polymorphism depends on several factors including the nature of the nucleotide variation, the local sequence of the gene, the possible availability of a restriction enzyme recognizing the sequence of one allele, cost of the detection method, etc. There are several in-house methods that have been published, while a number of kits made by private companies are available. In order to study a DNA polymorphism, molecular geneticists either sequence the gene region of interest or use a method involving polymerase chain reaction (PCR), followed by analysis of resulting DNA fragments by agarose gel electrophoresis.

The PCR method usually involves the following: (a) *simple use of a pair of primers,* if the two alleles differ in size, as in the case of the *ACE* I/D polymorphism; (b) *PCR followed by restriction enzyme,* if a restriction fragment length polymorphism (RFLP) is present, as in the case of *FV* Leiden (G1691A) in which endonuclease *TaqI* is used; (c) an *allele-specific primers,* when a common primer is coupled with each allele-specific oligonucleotide (ASO) primer in a separate PCR, as in the case of the *ITGA2* C807T polymorphism.

A typical PCR in total volume of 25–50 μl includes the following steps: (a) an initial denaturation step at 94°C for 4–5 min; (b) 30–35 cycles of a denaturation step at 94°C for 0.5–1 min, followed by an annealing step at primer-specific temperature for 0.5–1 min, followed by an elongation step at 72°C for 0.5–1 min; and (c) a final elongation step at 72°C for 5–7 min. Table 1 presents PCR annealing conditions and primers which may be used for the detection of functional DNA polymorphisms in thrombosis-related genes, using in-house protocols [11]. Table 2 mentions the expected sizes of DNA fragments viewed by agarose gel electrophoresis analysis.

Factor (gene polymorphism)	**Annealing temperature (°C)**	**Primers**	**Method**
Coagulation factors			
Coagulation factor II (F2 G20210A)	54	F: 5'-AACAACCGCTGGTATCAAATGG-3'	RFLP
		R: 5'-GAGCTGCCCATGAATAGCACTG-3'	
Coagulation factor V (F5 Leiden)	54	F: 5'-GCA GAT CCC TGG ACA GTC-3'	RFLP
		R: 5'-TGT TAT CAC ACT GGT GCT AA-3'	
Coagulation factor (FXII C46T)	57	F: 5'-ACTTCCAGGACCGCCTTTGGAGGC-3'	RFLP

http://dx.doi.org/10.5772/61859

Factor (gene polymorphism)	Annealing temperature (°C)	Primers	Method
		R: 5'-GTTGACGCCCCGGGGCACCG-3'	
Coagulation factor FXIII A1subunit (F13A1 V34L)	55	F: 5'-ACTTCCAGGACCGCCTTTGGAGGC-3'	RFLP
		R: 5'-GTTGACGCCCCGGGGCACCG-3'	
Fibrinolysis-related factors			
Serpine1 (PAI-1 4G/5G)	57	F: 5'- CACAGAGAGAGTCTGGCCACGT-3'	RFLP
		R: 5'-CCAACAGAGGACTCTTGGTCT-3'	
Plasma carboxypeptidase (CPB2, TAFI C1040T)	57	F: 5'-CACAAAGAAAAACAGATCACACAG-3'	RFLP
		R: 5'-AAAGCCACCCAATTGTGATT-3'	
Thrombin-related factors			
Thrombomodulin (THBD -13G/A)	58	F: 5'-ACCAAGAGATGAAAGAGGGC-3'	RFLP
		R: 5'-CGGATCGGCCAGGGCTCGAGTTTATAAAGGCC-3'	
Protein Z (PROZ -33A/G)	64	F: 5'-GGGTCCTCTGAGCCTTCACCGTTCATTT-3'	RFLP
		R: 5'-CAGGCACAACAGACAGGTAAGCCAGATG-3'	
Platelet-adhesion factors			
Intergin A2 (ITGA2, GPIA C807T)	56	COMMON: 5'-GACAGCCCATTAATAAATGTCTCCTCTG-3'	ASO
		C: 5'-CCTTGCATATTGAATTGCTACG-3'	
		T: 5'-CCTTGCATATTGAATTGCTACA-3'	
Platelet glycoprotein Iba (GPIBA VNTR)	63	F: 5'-ACACTTCACATGGACTCCAT--3'	VNTR
		R: 5'-GGGTCATTTCTGGAGCTCTC--3'	
Other factors			
Methylenetetrahydrofolate reductase(MTHFR C677T)	57	F: 5'-TGAAGGAGAAGGTGTCTGCGGGA-3'	RFLP
		R: 5'-AGGACGGTGCGGTGAGAGTG-3'	
Angiotensin I-converting enzyme (ACE I/D)	60	F: 5'-CTGGAGACCACTCCCATCCTTTCT-3'	PCR (I or D is amplified)
		R: 5'-GATGTGGCCATCACATTCGTCAGAT-3'	
		F1: 5'-TGGGACCACAGCGCCCGCCACTAC-3'	ASO (only I is amplified)
		R1: 5'-TCGCCAGCCCTCCCATGCCCATAA-3'	
Angiotensinogen (AGT M235T)	59	F: 5'-CAGGGTGCTGTCCACACTGGACCCC-3'	RFLP
		R: 5'-CCGTTTGTGCAGGGCCTGGCTCTCT-3'	

RFLP: restriction fragment length polymorphism; ASO: allele-specific oligonucleotide; VNTR: variable number tandem repeats.

Table 1. Conditions and primers which may be used for molecular detection of functional polymorphisms associated with thrombophilia.

Factor (gene polymorphism)	Method	Enzyme (Temperature, °C)	DNA fragments of normal allele (bp)	DNA fragments of variant allele (bp)
Coagulation factors				
Coagulation factor II (F2 G20210A))	RFLP	TaqI (65)	98 + 10	108
Coagulation factor V (F5 Leiden)	RFLP	TaqI (65)	157 + 18	175
Coagulation factor (FXII C46T))	RFLP	HgaI (37)	369	247 + 122
Coagulation factor FXIII A1subunit (F13A1 V34L)	RFLP	HhaI (37)	94 + 20	114
Fibrinolysis-related factors				
Fibrinolysis-related factors Serpine 1 (PAI-1 4G/5G)	RFLP	BslI (37)	77 + 22	99
Plasma carboxypeptidase (CPB2, TAFI C1040T)	RFLP	SpeI (37)	245 + 118	363
Thrombin-related factors				
Thrombomodulin (THBD -13G/A)	RFLP	StuI (37)	259	235 + 24
Protein Z (PROZ -33A/G)	RFLP	HhaI (37)	272	157 + 115
Platelet-adhesion factors				
Intergin A2 (ITGA2, GPIA C807T))	ASO		148	148
Platelet glycoprotein Iba (GPIBA VNTR)	VNTR		315, 237, 198	276
Other factors				
Methylenetetrajydrofolate reductase (MTHFR C677T)	RFLP	Hinf1 (37)	198	176 + 22
Angiotensin-converting enzyme (ACE I/D)	A ASO		190	490
Angiotensinogen(AGT M235T)	RFLP	TthIII (37)	165	141 + 24

RFLP: restriction fragment length polymorphism; ASO: allele-specific oligonucleotide; VNTR: variable number tandem repeats.

Table 2. DNA fragments observed after agarose gel electrophoresis.

11. Prevention of thrombosis

Individual susceptibility to thrombotic diseases, including venous thromboembolism, ischemic stroke and ischemic heart disorder, is known to be influenced by genetic factor in addition to lifestyle as reported in earlier studies [1–5, 10]. Prevention of idiopathic thrombosis is imperative, since it is very common and life-threatening [89–91]. Genetic counseling and presymptomatic DNA testing is especially important for people with a positive family history of thrombophilia. Several studies have indicated that pretest genetic counseling would be helpful in reducing anxiety and confusion about thrombophilia facts [10, 67, 92, 93]. Geneticists may play a significant role in the prevention of thrombophilia if, during their routine collection of family history data during counseling for other diseases, they recognize the individuals at risk for thrombosis and inform them about preventive measures, including the available molecular tests.

The ability to routinely detect the inherited genetic predisposition for thrombosis (either mutation- or disease-associated polymorphisms) may significantly contribute to early diagnosis and make possible early intervention and prevention of thrombotic incidents. Individuals with increased risk for thrombophilia should best be referred to hematologists who may advise some of them to receive preventive anticoagulant therapy. Particularly, women at risk for thrombosis should consult a hematologist before taking contraceptive pills, as well as in case of pregnancy. The optimal management of asymptomatic at risk individuals remains unclear, but it is generally agreed that thromboprophylaxis should be provided, at least in high-risk periods such as during surgery or pregnancy [10, 94–104].

Molecular diagnostics and prevention of thrombophilia will be greatly benefited when the relative contribution of each thrombosis-related DNA polymorphism to vascular disease is better understood, possibly with the aid of large-scale epidemiological studies. Only then, a population-wide screening might be warranted for preventative purposes. At this stage, initial information about the prevalence of major DNA polymorphisms is recommended for each population in order to shape local health policies for prevention of thrombosis by identification of individuals at risk.

As an example, in southern and eastern Europeans prevention of thrombophilia may be significantly effected by studying genetic variants *FV* Leiden and *FII* G20210A since they both appear to be found in relatively high frequencies and to be major susceptibility factors for thromboembolic incidents in these populations [55, 67, 105–110]. A study in Greeks indicated that the combination of genetic counseling and molecular testing for these two common thrombophilia may increase up to fivefold the identification of at risk individuals compared to population-wide screening and has a significant impact on the prevention of thromboembolic incidents [66].

As genetic testing becomes a routine approach, it is expected that it will be extensively used both in hospital and community preventive medicine. Accordingly, it may be envisaged that thrombophilia, which is currently such a major global burden, shall be routinely preventable in the future with the aid of genetic testing and proper anticoagulant treatment, thus safeguarding the life and health status of asymptomatic individuals at risk.

Acknowledgements

The authors would like to cordially thank Dr. Thalia Antoniadi for helpful discussions in initial stage of thrombophilia research. This text is dedicated to Professor Emeritus of Internal Medicine and Hematology Dimitris Loukopoulos.

Author details

Christos Yapijakis*, Zoe Serefoglou and Constantinos Voumvourakis

*Address all correspondence to: cyapijakis_ua_gr@yahoo.com

Department of Neurology, University of Athens Medical School, Athens, Greece

References

[1] Lozano R, Naghavi M, Foreman K et al. Global and regional mortality from 235 cases of death for 20 age groups in 1990 and 2010. Lancet. 2012;380:2095–2128.

[2] Raskob GE, Angchaisuksiri P, Blanco AN et al. Thrombosis: A major contributor to the global disease burden. J Thromb Haemost. 2014;12:1580–1590.

[3] Albisetti M, Moeller A, Waldvogel K, Bernet-Buettiker V, Cannizzaro V, Anagnostopoulos A, Balmer C and Schmugge M. Congenital prothrombotic disorders in children with peripheral venous and arterial thromboses. Acta Haematol. 2007;117:149–155.

[4] Bick RL. Hereditary and acquired thrombophilic disorders. Clin Appl Thromb Hemost. 2006;12:125–135.

[5] Gary T, Hafner F, Froehlich H, Stojakovic T, Scharnagl H, Pilger E and Brodmann M. High factor VIII activity, high plasminogen activator inhibitor 1 antigen levels and low factor XII activity contribute to a thrombophilic tendency in elderly venous thromboembolism patients. Acta Haematol. 2010;124:214–217.

[6] Banerjee I, Gupta V and Ganesh S. Association of gene polymorphism with genetic susceptibility to stroke in Asian populations: A meta-analysis. J Hum Genet. 2007;52:205–219.

[7] Kim RJ and Becker RC. Association between factor V Leiden, prothrombin G20210A, and methylene tetrahydrofolate reductase C677T mutations and events of the arterial circulatory system: A meta-analysis of published studies. Am Heart J. 2003;146:948–957.

[8] Klerk M, Verhoef P, Clarke R, Blom HJ, Kok FJ and Schouten EG: MTHFR 677C>T polymorphism and risk of coronary heart disease: A meta-analysis. JAMA. 2002;288:2023–2031.

[9] Lane DA and Grant PJ: Role of hemostatic gene polymorphisms in venous and arterial thrombotic disease. Blood. 2000;95:1517–1532.

[10] Reitsma PH. Genetics in thrombophilia. An update. Hämostaseologie. 2015;35:47–51.

[11] Yapijakis C, Serefoglou Z, Nixon AM, Vylliotis A, Ragos V, Vairaktaris E. Prevalence of thrombosis- related DNA polymorphisms in a healthy Greek population. In Vivo. 2012;26:1095–1102.

[12] Nash GF, Walsh DC and Kakkar AK: The role of the coagulation system in tumour angiogenesis. Lancet Oncol. 2001;2:608–613.

[13] Gomez K and McVey JH: Tissue factor initiated blood coagulation. Front Biosci. 2006;11:1349–1359.

[14] Peppelenbosch MP and Versteeg HH: Cell biology of tissue factor, an unusual member of the cytokine receptor family. Trends Cardiovasc Med. 2001;11:335–339.

[15] Crawley JT and Lane DA: The haemostatic role of tissue factor pathway inhibitor. Arterioscler Thromb Vasc Biol. 2008;28(2):233–242.

[16] Carmeliet P, Ferreira V, Breier G, Pollefeyt S, Kieckens L, Gertsenstein M, Fahrig M, Vandenhoeck A, Harpal K, Eberhardt C, Declercq C, Pawling J, Moons L, Collen D, Risau W and Nagy A: Abnormal blood vessel development and lethality in embryos lacking a single *VEGF* allele. Nature. 1996;380:435–439.

[17] Olivier V, Bentolila S, Chabbat J, Hakim J and de Prost D: Tissue factor-dependent vascular endothelial growth factor production by human fibroblasts in response to activated factor VII. Blood. 1998;91:2698–2703.

[18] Taniguchi T, Kakkar AK, Tuddenham EG, Williamson RC and Lemoine NR: Enhanced expression of urokinase receptor induced through the tissue factor-factor VIIa pathway in human pancreatic cancer. Cancer Res. 1998;58:4461–4467.

[19] Mechtcheriakova D, Wlachos A, Holzmuller, Binder BR and Hofer E: Vascular endothelial cell growth factor-induced tissue factor expression in endothelial cells is mediated by EGR-1. Blood. 1999;93:3811–3823.

[20] Yapijakis C, Vairaktaris E, Vassiliou S, Vylliotis A, Nkenke E, Nixon AM, Derka S, Spyridonidou S, Vorris E, Neukam F and Patsouris E: The low VEGF production allele of the +936C/T polymorphism is strongly associated with increased risk for oral cancer. J Cancer Res Clin Oncol. 2007;133:787–791.

[21] Coughlin SR: Thrombin signalling and protease-activated receptors. Nature. 2000;407:258–264.

[22] Maragoudakis ME, Kraniti N, Giannopoulou E, Alexopoulos K and Matsoukas J: Modulation of angiogenesis and progelatinase a by thrombin receptor mimetics and antagonists. Endothelium. 2001;8:195–205.

[23] Tsopanoglou NE and Maragoudakis ME: On the mechanism of thrombin-induced angiogenesis. Potentiation of vascular endothelial growth factor activity on endothelial cells by upregulation of its receptors. J Biol Chem. 1999;274:23969–23976.

[24] Tsopanoglou NE, Andriopoulou P and Maragoudakis ME: On the mechanism of thrombin-induced angiogenesis: Involvement of $\alpha v\beta 3$-integrin. Am J Physiol Cell Physiol. 2002;283:1501–1510.

[25] Tsopanoglou NE and Maragoudakis ME: Role of thrombin in angiogenesis and tumor progression. Semin Thromb Hemost. 2004;30:63–69.

[26] Lee TH, Rhim T and Kim SS: Prothrombin kringle-2 domain has a growth inhibitory activity against basic fibroblast growth factor-stimulated capillary endothelial cells. J Biol Chem. 1998;273:28805–28812.

[27] Rhim TY, Park CS, Kim E and Kim SS: Human prothrombin fragment 1 and 2 inhibit bFGF-induced BCE cell growth. Biochem Biophys Res Commun. 1998;252:513–516.

[28] Bouma BN and Mosnier LO: Thrombin activatable fibrinolysis inhibitor (TAFI) – How does thrombin regulate fibrinolysis? Ann Med. 2006;38:378–388.

[29] Koutsi A, Papapanagiotou A and Papavassiliou AG: Thrombomodulin: From haemostasis to inflammation and tumourigenesis. Int J Biochem Cell Biol. 2008;40:1669–1673.

[30] Mosesson MW: Fibrinogen and fibrin structure and functions. J Thromb Haemost. 2005;3:1894–1904.

[31] Fernandez PM, Patierno SR and Rickles FR: Tissue factor and fibrin in tumor angiogenesis. Semin Thromb Hemost. 2004;30:31–44.

[32] Sahni A, Simpson-Haidaris PJ, Sahni SK, Vaday GG and Francis CW: Fibrinogen synthesized by cancer cells augments the proliferative effect of FGF-2. J Thromb Haemost. 2008;6:176–183.

[33] Dvorak HF: Tumors: Wounds that do not heal. Similarities between tumor stroma generation and wound healing. N Engl J Med. 1986;315:1650–1659.

[34] Dvorak HF: Rous-Whipple Award Lecture. How tumors make bad blood vessels and stroma. Am J Pathol. 2003;162:1747–1757.

[35] Engelse MA, Hanemaaijer R, Koolwijk P and van Hinsbergh VW: The fibrinolytic system and matrix metalloproteinases in angiogenesis and tumor progression. Semin Thromb Hemost. 2004;30:71–82.

[36] Wojtukiewicz MZ, Sierko E and Rak J: Contribution of the hemostatic system to angiogenesis in cancer. Semin Thromb Hemost. 2004;30:5–20.

[37] Nakasaki T, Wada H, Shigemori C, Miki C, Gabazza EC, Nobori T, Nakamura S and Shiku H: Expression of tissue factor and vascular endothelial growth factor is associated with angiogenesis in colorectal cancer. Am J Hematol. 2002;69:247–254.

[38] Shoji M, Hancock WW, Abe K, Micko C, Casper KA, Baine RM, Wilcox JN, Danave I, Dillehay DL, Matthews E, Contrino J, Morrissey JH, Gordon S, Edgington TS, Kudryk B, Kreutzer DL and Rickles FR: Activation of coagulation and angiogenesis in cancer: Immunohistochemical localization *in situ* of clotting proteins and vascular endothelial growth factor in human cancer. Am J Pathol. 1998;152:399–411.

[39] Tsigris C, Chatzitheofylaktou A, Xiromeritis C, Nikiteas N and Yannopoulos A: Genetic association studies in digestive system malignancies. Anticancer Res. 2007;27(5B):3577–3587.

[40] Vairaktaris E, Serefoglou Z, Avgoustidis D, Yapijakis C, Critselis E, Vylliotis A, Spyridonidou S, Derka S, Vassiliou S, Nkenke E and Patsouris E: Gene polymorphisms related to angiogenesis, inflammation and thrombosis that influence risk for oral cancer. Oral Oncol. 2009;45:247–253.

[41] Franchini M, Montagnana M, Targher G, Manzato F and Lippi G: Pathogenesis, clinical and laboratory aspects of thrombosis in cancer. J Thromb Thrombolysis. 2007;24:29–38.

[42] De Cicco M: The prothrombotic state in cancer: Pathogenic mechanisms. Crit Rev Oncol Hematol. 2004;50:187–196.

[43] Falanga A, Panova-Noeva M and Russo L: Procoagulant mechanisms in tumour cells. Best Pract Res Clin Haematol. 2009;22:49–60.

[44] Elice F, Jacoub J, Rickles FR, Falanga and Liebman HA: Hemostatic complications of angiogenesis inhibitors in cancer patients. Am J Hematol. 2008;83:862–870.

[45] Sutherland DE, Weitz IC and Liebman HA: Thromboembolic complications of cancer: Epidemiology, pathogenesis, diagnosis, and treatment. Am J Hematol. 2003;72:43–52.

[46] Wünsch Filho V and Zago MA: Modern cancer epidemiological research: Genetic polymorphisms and environment. Rev Saude Publica. 2005;39(3):490–497.

[47] Hirschhorn JN, Lohmueller Kirk, Byrne E and Hirschhorn K: A comprehensive review of genetic association studies. Genet Med. 2002;4(2):45–61.

[48] Cooper DN, Nussbaum RL and Krawczak M: Proposed guidelines for papers describing DNA polymorphism-disease associations. Hum Genet. 2002;110(3):207–208.

[49] Guo SW and Thompson EA: Performing the exact test of Hardy-Weinberg proportion for multiple alleles. Biometrics. 1992;48:361–372.

[50] Vairaktaris E, Yapijakis C, Serefoglou Z, Avgoustidis D, Critselis E, Spyridonidou S, Vylliotis A, Derka S, Vassiliou S, Nkenke E and Patsouris E: Gene expression polymorphisms of interleukins-1beta, -4, -6, -8, -10, and tumor necrosis factors alpha, -beta: Regression analysis of their effect upon oral squamous cell carcinoma. J Cancer Res Clin Oncol. 2008;134:821–832.

[51] Ageno W, Squizzato A, Garcia D and Imberti D: Epidemiology and risk factors of venous thromboembolism. Semin Thromb Hemost. 2006;32:651–658.

[52] Musunuru K and Kathiresan S: HapMap and mapping genes for cardiovascular disease. Circ Cardiovasc Genet. 2008;1:66–71.

[53] Hoppe B, Tolou F, Dorner T, Kiesewetter H and Salama A: Gene polymorphisms implicated in influencing susceptibility to venous and arterial thromboembolism: Frequency distribution in a healthy German population. Thromb Haemost. 2006;96:465–470.

[54] Ireland H, Kunz G, Kyriakoulis K, Stubbs PJ and Lane DA: Thrombomodulin gene mutations associated with myocardial infarction. Circulation. 1997;96:15–18.

[55] Koumas L, Costeas PA, Papaloizou A and Giantsiou-Kyriakou A: Genetic assessment of cardiovascular risk factors in the Greek Cypriot population. Thromb Res. 2003;112:143–146.

[56] Martini CH, Doggen CJ, Cavallini C, Rosendaal FR and Mannucci PM: No effect of polymorphisms in prothrombotic genes on the risk of myocardial infarction in young adults without cardiovascular risk factors. J Thromb Haemost. 2005;3:177–179.

[57] Vairaktaris E, Yapijakis C, Serefoglou Z, Vylliotis A, Ries J, Nkenke E, Wiltfang J, Derka S, Vassiliou S, Springer I, Kessler P and Neukam FW: Plasminogen activator inhibitor-1 polymorphism is associated with increased risk for oral cancer. Oral Oncol. 2006;42:888–892.

[58] Zama T, Murata M, Ono F, Watanabe K, Watanabe R, Moriki T, Yokoyama K, Tokuhira M and Ikeda Y: Low prevalence of activated protein C resistance and coagulation factor V Arg506 to Gln mutation among Japanese patients with various forms of thrombosis, and normal individuals. Int J Hematol. 1996;65:71–78.

[59] Zhao J, Zhou X, Huang J, Chen J and Gu D: Association study of the thrombomodulin –33G>A polymorphism with coronary artery disease and myocardial infarction in Chinese Han population. Int J Cardiol. 2005;100:383–388.

[60] Bauduer F and Lacombe D: Factor V Leiden, prothrombin 20210A, methylene tetrahydrofolate reductase 677T, and population genetics. Mol Genet Metab. 2005;86:91–99.

[61] Bertina RM: Factor V Leiden and other coagulation factor mutations affecting thrombotic risk. Clin Chem. 1997;43:1678–1684.

[62] Coppage KH, Hinton AC, Moldenhauer J, Kovilam O, Barton JR and Sibai BM: Maternal and perinatal outcome in women with a history of stroke. Am J Obstet Gynecol. 2004;190:1331–1334.

[63] Foka ZJ, Lambropoulos AF, Saravelos H, Karas GB, Karavida A, Agorastos T, Zournatzi V, Makris PE, Bontis J and Kotsis A: Factor V leiden and prothrombin G20210A mutations, but not methylene tetrahydrofolate reductase C677T, are associated with recurrent miscarriages. Hum Reprod. 2000;15:458–462.

[64] Ridker PM, Hennekens CH, Lindpainter K, Stampfer MJ, Eisenberg PR and Miletich JP: Mutation in the gene coding for coagulation factor V and the risk of myocardial infarction, stroke, and venous thrombosis in apparently healthy men. N Engl J Med. 1995;332:912–917.

[65] Yapijakis C, Antoniadi T, Salavoura K, Voumvourakis C and Vairaktaris E: Potential prevention of thromboembolism by genetic counseling and testing for two common thrombophilia mutations. In Vivo. 2012;26:165–172.

[66] De Stefano V, Martinelli I, Mannucci PM, Paciaroni K, Chiusolo P, Casorelli I, Rossi E, and Leone G: The risk of recurrent deep venous thrombosis among heterozygous carriers of both factor V Leiden and the G20210A prothrombin mutation. N Engl J Med. 1999;341:801–806.

[67] Poort SR, Rosendaal FR, Reitsma PH and Bertina RM: A common genetic variation in the 3'-untranslated region of the prothrombin gene is associated with elevated plasma prothrombin levels and an increase in venous thrombosis. Blood. 1996;88:3698–3703.

[68] Santamaria A, Mateo J, Tirado I, Oliver A, Belvis R, Marti-Fabregas J, Felices R, Soria JM, Souto JC and Fontcuberta J: Homozygosity of the T allele of the 46 C/T polymorphism in the F12 gene is a risk factor for ischemic stroke in the Spanish population. Stroke. 2004;35:1795–1799.

[69] Wells PS, Anderson JL, Scarvelis DK, Doucette SP and Gagnon F: Factor XIII Val34Leu variant is protective against venous thromboembolism: A HuGE review and meta-analysis. Am J Epidemiol. 2006;164:101–109.

[70] Cesari F, Fatini C, Sticchi E, Fedi S, Abbate R, Gensini GF and Sofi F: Protein Z gene polymorphisms (intron F 79 G>A; –13A>G) are not associated with acute coronary syndromes. Thromb Haemost. 2006;96:98–99.

[71] Eriksson P, Kallin B, van't Hooft FM, Bavenholm P and Hamsten A: Allele-specific increase in basal transcription of the plasminogen-activator inhibitor 1 gene is associated with myocardial infarction. Proc Natl Acad Sci U S A. 1995;92:1851–1855.

[72] Grubic N, Stegnar M, Peternel P, Kaider A and Binder BR: A novel G/A and the 4G/5G polymorphism within the promoter of the plasminogen activator inhibitor-1 gene in patients with deep vein thrombosis. Thromb Res. 1996;84:431–443.

[73] Morange PE, Tregouet DA, Frere C, Luc G, Arveiler D, Ferrieres J, Amouyel P, Evans A, Ducimetiere P, Cambien F, Tiret L and Juhan-Vague I; Prime Study Group: TAFI gene haplotypes, TAFI plasma levels and future risk of coronary heart disease: The PRIME Study. J Thromb Haemost. 2005;3:1503–1510.

[74] Schneider M, Boffa M, Stewart R et al. Two naturally occurring variants of TAFI (Thr-325 and Ile-325) differ substantially with respect to thermal stability and antifibrinolytic activity of the enzyme. J Biol Chem. 2002;277:1021–1030.

[75] Ozelo MC, Origa AF, Aranha FJ, Mansur AP, Annichino-Bizzacchi JM, Costa FF, Pollak ES and Arruda VR: Platelet glycoprotein Ib alpha polymorphisms modulate the risk for myocardial infarction. Thromb Haemost. 2004;92:384–386.

[76] Wagner C and Bailey LB (eds): Folate in health and disease. Marcel Dekker, New York, 1995.

[77] Frosst P, Blom HJ, Milos R, Goyette P, Sheppard CA, Matthews RG, Boers GJ, den Heijer M, Kluijtmans LA and van den Heuvel LP: A candidate genetic risk factor for vascular disease: A common mutation in methylenetetrahydrofolate reductase. Nat Genet. 1995;10:111–113.

[78] Goracy I, Cyrylowski L, Kaczmarczyk M, Fabian A, Koziarska D, Goracy J and Ciechanowicz A: C677T polymorphism of the methylene tetrahydrofolate reductase gene and the risk of ischemic stroke in Polish subjects. J Appl Genet. 2009;50:63–67.

[79] Jacques PF, Bostom AG, Williams RR, Ellison RC, Eckfeldt JH, Rosenberg IH, Selhub J and Rosen R: Relation between folate status, a common mutation in methylenetetrahydrofolate reductase, and plasma homocysteine concentrations. Circulation. 1996;93:7–9.

[80] Gudnason V, Stansbie D, Scott J, Browron A, Nicaud V and Humphries S. C677T (thermolabile alanine/valine) polymorphism in methylenetetrahydrofolate reductase (MTHFR): its frequency and impact on plasma homocysteine concentration in different European populations. Atherosclerosis. 1998;136:347–354.

[81] Stroth U and Unger T. The renin angiotensin system and its receptors. J Cardiovasc Pharmacol. 1999;33:21–28.

[82] Caulfield M, Lavender P, Farrall M, Munroe P, Lawson M, Turner P and Clark AJ: Linkage of the angiotensinogen gene to essential hypertension. N Engl J Med. 1994;330:1629–1633.

[83] Hata A, Namikawa C, Sasaki M, Sato K, Nakamura T, Tamura K and Lalouel JM: Angiotensinogen as a risk factor for essential hypertension in Japan. J Clin Invest. 1994;93:1285–1287.

[84] Hegele RA, Brunt JH and Connelly PW: A polymorphism of the angiotensinogen gene associated with variation in blood pressure in a genetic isolate. Circulation. 1994;90:2207–2212.

[85] Jeunemaitre X, Soubrier F, Kotelevtsev YV, Lifton RP, Williams CS, Charru A, Hunt SC, Hopkins PN, Williams RR, Lalouel JM et al: Molecular basis of human hypertension: role of angiotensinogen. Cell. 71:7–20.

[86] Staessen J, Kuznetsova T, Wang J, Emelianov D, Vlietinck R and Fagard R: M235T angiotensinogen gene polymorphism and cardiovascular renal risk. J Hypertens. 1999;17:9–17.

[87] Zhu X, McKenzie CA, Forrester T, Nickerson DA, Broeckel U and Schunkert H et al. Localization of a small genomic region associated with elevated ACE. Am J Hum Genet. 2000;67:1144–1153.

[88] McKenzie CA, Julier C, Forrester T, McFarlane-Anderson N, Keavney B, Lathrop GM et al. Segregation and linkage analysis of serum angiotensin I-converting enzyme levels: Evidence for two quantitative-trait loci. Am J Hum Genet. 1995;57:1426–1435.

[89] Bang SM, Jang MJ, Kim KH, Yhim HY, Kim YK, Nam SH, Hwang HG, Bae SH, Kim SH, Mun YC, Kim YK, Kim I, Choi WI, Jung CW, Park NH, Choi NK, Park BJ and Oh D: Prevention of Venous Thromboembolism, 2nd Edition: Korean Society of Thrombosis and Hemostasis Evidence-Based Clinical Practice Guidelines. Korean Med Sci. 2014;29:164–171.

[90] Cardiovascular Disease Educational and Research Trust, Cyprus Cardiovascular Disease Educational and Research Trust, European Venous Forum, International Surgical Thrombosis Forum, International Union of Angiology, Union Internationale de Phlébologie: Prevention and treatment of venous thromboembolism: International Consensus Statement (guidelines according to scientific evidence). Int Angiol. 2006;25:101–161.

[91] Guyatt GH, Akl EA, Crowther M, Gutterman DD, Schuünemann HJ, American College of Chest Physicians Antithrombotic Therapy and Prevention of Thrombosis Panel: Executive summary: Antithrombotic therapy and prevention of thrombosis, 9th ed: American College of Chest Physicians Evidence-Based Clinical Practice Guidelines. Chest. 1012;141:7S-47S.

[92] Federici C, Gianetti J and Andreassi MG: Genomic medicine and thrombotic risk: Who, when, how and why? Int J Cardiol. 2006;106:3–9.

[93] Reich LM, Bower M and Keys NS. Role of the geneticist in testing and counseling for inherited thrombophilia. Genet Med. 2003;5:133–143.

[94] Coppens M, van de Poel MH, Bank I, Hamulyak K, van der Meer J, Veeger NJ, Prins MH, Buller HR and Middeldorp S: A prospective cohort study on the absolute incidence of venous thromboembolism and arterial cardiovascular disease in asymptomatic carriers of the prothrombin 20210A mutation. Blood. 2006;108:2604–2607.

[95] de Maistre E, Terriat B, Lesne-Padieu AS, Abello N, Bouchot O and Steinmetz EF: High incidence of venous thrombosis after surgery for abdominal aortic aneurysm. J Vasc Surg. 2009;49:596–601.

[96] Horne MK 3rd and McCloskey DJ: Factor V Leiden as a common genetic risk factor for venous thromboembolism. J Nurs Scholarsh. 2006;38:19–25.

[97] Kakkos SK, Sabetai M, Tegos T, Stevens J, Thomas D, Griffin M, Geroulakos G and Nicolaides AN: Asymptomatic Carotid Stenosis and Risk of Stroke (ACSRS) Study Group: Silent embolic infarcts on computed tomography brain scans and risk of ipsilateral hemispheric events in patients with asymptomatic internal carotid artery stenosis. J Vasc Surg. 2009;49:902–909.

[98] King A and Markus HS: Doppler embolic signals in cerebrovascular disease and prediction of stroke risk: A systematic review and meta-analysis. Stroke. 2009;40:3711–3717.

[99] Langlois NJ and Wells PS: Risk of venous thromboembolism in relatives of symptomatic probands with thrombophilia: A systematic review. Thromb Haemost. 2003;90:17–26.

[100] Said JM, Higgins JR, Moses EK, Walker SP, Borg AJ, Monagle PT and Brennecke SP: Inherited thrombophilia polymorphisms and pregnancy outcomes in outcomes in nulliparous women. Obstet Gynecol. 2010;115:5–13.

[101] Selby R, Geerts W, Ofosu FA, Craven S, Dewar L, Phillips A and Szalai JP: Hypercoagulability after trauma: Hemostatic changes and relationship to venous thromboembolism. Thromb Res. 2009;124:281–287.

[102] Simioni P, Tormene D, Prandoni P, Zerbinati P, Gavasso S, Cefalo P and Girolami A: Incidence of venous thromboembolism in asymptomatic family members who are carriers of factor V Leiden: A prospective cohort study. Blood. 2002;99:1938–1942.

[103] Taniguchi S, Fukuda I, Daitoku K, Minakawa M, Odagiri S, Suzuki Y, Fukui K, Asano K and Ohkuma H: Prevalence of venous thromboembolism in neurosurgical patients. Heart Vessels. 2009;24:425–428.

[104] Zubkov AY and Wijdicks EF: Deep venous thrombosis prophylaxis in cerebral hemorrhage. Rev Neurol Dis. 2009;6:21–25.

[105] Antoniades C, Tousoulis D, Vasiliadou C, Stefanadi E, Marinou K and Stefanadis C: Genetic polymorphisms of platelet glycoprotein Ia and the risk for premature myocardial infarction: Effects on the release of sCD40L during the acute phase of premature myocardial infarction. J Am Coll Cardiol. 2006;47:1959–1966.

[106] Antoniadi T, Hatzis T, Kroupis C, Economou-Petersen E and Petersen MB: Prevalence of factor V Leiden, prothrombin G20210A, and *MTHFR* C677T mutations in a Greek population of blood donors. Am J Hematol. 1999;61:265–267.

[107] Chaida C, Gialeraki A, Tsoukala C and Mandalaki T: Prevalence of the FVQ506 mutation in the Hellenic population. Thromb Haemost. 1996;76:127.

[108] Ioannou HV, Mitsis M, Eleftheriou A, Matsagas M, Nousias V, Rigopoulos C, Vartholomatos G and Kappas AM: The prevalence of factor V Leiden as a risk factor for venous thromboembolism in the population of North-Western Greece. Int Angiol. 2000;19:314–318.

[109] Vassilikioti S, Doumas M, Douma S, Petidis K, Karagiannis A, Balaska K, Vyzantiadis A and Zamboulis C: Angiotensin converting enzyme gene polymorphism is not related to essential hypertension in a Greek population. Am J Hypertens. 1996;9:700–702.

[110] Xenophontos SL, Hadjivassiliou M, Ayrton N, Karagrigoriou A, Pantzaris M, Nicolaides AN and Cariolou MA: Spectrum and prevalence of prothrombotic single nucleotide polymorphism profiles in the Greek Cypriot population. Int Angiol. 2002;21:322–329.

Chapter 6

Laboratory Methodology Important in the Diagnosis and Prognosis of Antiphospholipid Syndrome

Polona Žigon, Mojca Božič-Mijovski, Mojca Frank Bertoncelj, Aleš Ambrožič, Matija Tomšič, Alojzija Hočevar, Borut Božič, Snežna Sodin Šemrl, Tanja Kveder and Saša Čučnik

Additional information is available at the end of the chapter

http://dx.doi.org/10.5772/61551

Abstract

Antiphospholipid syndrome (APS) is an autoimmune disease, characterized by thrombosis and pregnancy complications with persistently elevated levels of antiphospholipid antibodies (aPL). Recently, a unique mathematical calculation has been presented to assess the risk of thrombosis in patients with APS called antiphospholipid score or global antiphospholipid syndrome score (GAPSS). This new approach in the diagnosis of APS leads to the assessment of the risk of thrombosis considering the results of different aPL (lupus anticoagulants (LA), anticardiolipin antibodies (aCL), antibodies against β2GPI (anti-β2GPI), and phosphatidylserine-dependent antiprothrombin antibodies (aPS/PT) (isotypes IgG and IgM). This chapter provides an overview of the algorithm strategy for APS diagnosis with the aims of characterizing in detail the laboratory methodology of criteria aPL (LA, aCL, and anti-β2GPI) and noncriteria aPL, such as IgA aCL and IgA anti-β2GPI, anti-domain I β2GPI, and antiprothrombin antibodies. In order to improve APS diagnosis, several new approaches in aPL detection have recently been suggested, such as multiline immunodot assay, detection of aPL by flow cytometry using beads with particular surface properties, and the newly developed automated BioPlex system technology for parallel detection of aCL and anti-β2GPI antibodies of IgG, IgA, and IgM isotypes. A completely different and promising approach in future research lies in the potential of microRNAs as biomarkers for risk of thrombosis and/or obstetric complication.

Keywords: Anticardiolipin antibodies, lupus anticoagulants, anti-beta2-glycoprotein I antibodies, antiprothrombin antibodies, ELISA, multiplex assays, microRNA studies

1. Introduction

The antiphospholipid syndrome (APS) or Hughes syndrome was first described three decades ago in patients with systemic lupus erythematosus and positive pathogenic autoantibodies named antiphospholipid antibodies (aPL), who experienced arterial or venous thrombosis [1]. APS is now recognized as an autoimmune disease, characterized by thrombosis and pregnancy complications with persistently elevated levels of aPL. While deep veins of the lower limbs and the cerebral arterial circulation are the most common sites of venous and arterial thrombosis, any tissue or organ can be affected [2]. The risk of recurrent thrombosis in APS over 5 years is 16.6% despite the use of anticoagulants and/or salicylates [3, 4]. APS is also associated with a 5-year mortality of 5.3% with most deaths occurring within the first year of diagnosis due prevalently to bacterial infections, myocardial infarction, stroke, and cerebral hemorrhage [5]. The catastrophic APS (CAPS) is a rare life-threatening form of APS in which widespread intravascular thrombosis results in multiorgan ischemia and failure. Intravascular thrombosis affecting predominantly microcirculation characterizes CAPS. In addition, thrombosis of arteries, veins, or both can occur. CAPS affects about 1% of cases with APS and is the initial presentation of APS in nearly half of patients, while the remaining half has a history of APS [6–9]. Despite aggressive treatment, mortality rates still range between 44.0% and 55.6% [5, 10]. The other major clinical manifestations of APS are obstetrical. They include the unexplained death of one or more morphologically normal fetuses at or beyond the 10th week of gestation, the premature birth of one or more morphologically normal neonates before the 34th week of gestation due to eclampsia, severe preeclampsia, or recognized features of placental insufficiency, and three or more unexplained consecutive spontaneous abortions before the 10th week of gestation.

According to the international consensus statement on classification criteria established in 1999 in Sapporo and updated in 2006 in Sydney, APS is classified when persistently elevated levels of specific aPL are confirmed in addition to clinical manifestations [11, 12]. These consensus classification criteria for definite APS enabled substantial improvement in APS recognition (Figure 1); however, the diagnosis of APS still remains difficult. In the general population, the incidence of clinical manifestations which can be included in APS is high and could often be triggered by other underlying factors. Consequently, the diagnosis of APS relies predominantly on the laboratory results. The laboratory criteria comprise persistently elevated levels of either lupus anticoagulant (LA) or IgG/IgM antibodies to cardiolipin (aCL) or antibodies to β_2GPI (anti-β_2GPI). Methods for their determination differ and have not yet been standardized [13]. The common weaknesses of aPL determination are high interassay and interlaboratory variations, problems with the interpretation and clinical evaluation of the test results, as well as their low diagnostic specificity. Elevated aPL can be associated with many other conditions such as infections, malignancy, and also exposure to certain drugs. The absence of reliable, robust diagnostic markers for APS thus limits patient identification and management which challenges researchers to find better diagnostic marker(s). Among many autoantibodies that have been found to be associated with APS but not included in the current laboratory criteria, antiprothrombin antibodies have shown the highest diagnostic applicability. Moreover, antiprothrombin antibodies are often present in APS patients and are sometimes the only aPL elevated [14, 15]. A recently published review concluded that an immunoassay using phosphatidylserine/prothrombin (aPS/PT ELISA) as an antigen on solid phase, leads to higher diagnostic accuracy as compared to the method using prothrombin alone (aPT ELISA) [14]. It seems that in the future there might be a change in the perception of the role of aPL from the criterion for APS classification to the role of risk factors estimating the probability for developing APS clinical manifestation. Modern trends for the diagnostic evaluation of APS patients therefore propose a determination of multiple classes of aPL, among them also antiprothrombin antibodies, to gain a common score which estimates the risk for arterial/venous thrombosis in APS patients [16–18]. Risk stratification is a major challenge in treating patients with APS and a potential role of aPL as a risk or even as a prognostic factor for arterial/venous thrombosis and miscarriages has been intensively debated [16, 19]. Single, double, and triple aPL positivity is not rare in patients with APS and such multiple positivity is mostly associated with higher risk for appearance or recurrence of thrombotic events and miscarriages [20, 21]. Recently, two research groups presented a unique mathematical calculation to assess the risk of thrombosis in patients with APS (called antiphospholipid score or global antiphospholipid syndrome score-GAPSS) [16, 17]. This new approach in the diagnosis of APS leads to the assessment of the risk of thrombosis considering the results of different aPL (LA, aCL, anti-β_2GPI, and aPS/PT—isotypes IgG and IgM). The common calculation can help clinicians decide about introducing, eliminating or changing the appropriate therapy.

In order to improve APS diagnosis, several new approaches in aPL detection have recently been suggested. One is to detect aPL antibodies by multiline immunodot assay which may provide an interesting alternative to ELISA. Multiline immunodot assay could be a candidate for an effective multiparameter test system and simultaneous, semi-quantitative detection of several aPL antibodies in one sample; however, the technique has not yet been widely studied [22]. Apart from the immunodot technique, the detection of aPL by flow cytometry using beads with particular surface properties could represent another promising approach in aPL antibody multiplex testing [23]. Very recently, an automated technology for the parallel detection of aCL and anti-β_2GPI antibodies of IgG, IgA, and IgM isotypes was developed in the BioPlex system [24]. The instrument combines the multianalyte profiling technology with antigen-coated fluoromagnetic beads in an automated platform where sampling, processing, and data reduction are performed automatically.

A completely different and promising approach in future research lies in the potential added value of microRNAs (miRNAs) as biomarkers for risk of thrombosis and/or obstetric complication. These are small noncoding RNAs that regulate gene expression at the posttranscriptional level by degrading or blocking translation of messenger RNAs. Many miRNAs have been found significantly altered in sera or plasma of patients with thrombosis [25] or specific pregnancy complications [26, 27].

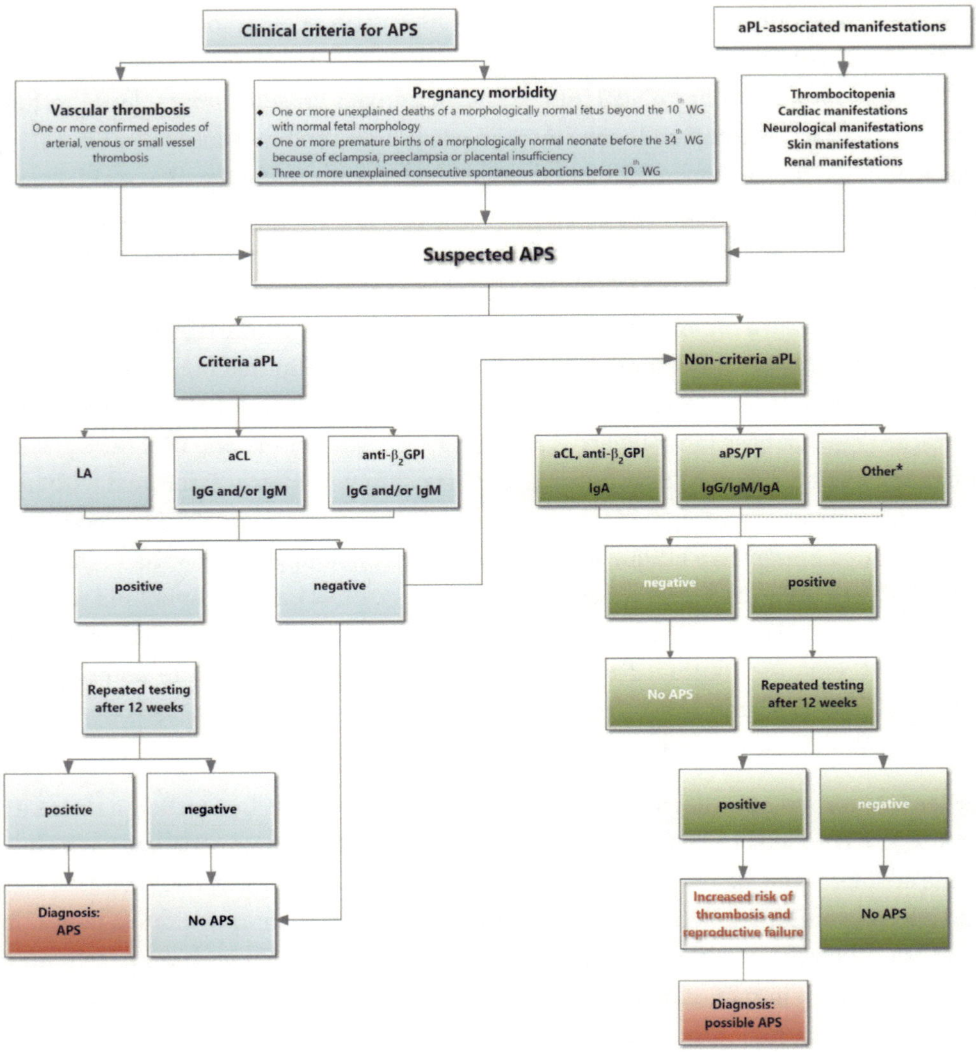

*Anti-annexin V antibodies, anti-phosphatidylethanolamine, antibodies to domains of β_2GPI, antibodies against anionic phospholipids other than cardiolipin [28, 29].

Figure 1. Algorithm strategy for APS diagnosis. APS: antiphospholipid syndrome; aCL: anticardiolipin antibodies, anti-β_2GPI: antibodies against β_2 glycoprotein I; aPS/PT: antiphosphatidylserine prothrombin antibodies; aPL: antiphospholipid antibodies, LA: lupus anticoagulant.

2. Criteria aPL

Despite several attempts to standardize the LA, aCL, and anti-β_2GPI tests, a considerable degree of interlaboratory variation still exists [13, 30]. While many laboratories worldwide

http://dx.doi.org/10.5772/61551

have managed to obtain consistently reproducible LA, aCL, and anti-β_2GPI results, there are others that still report variations between different runs, which may potentially affect the consistency of the diagnosis of APS. This is mainly due to laboratories performing in-house aPL assays or using commercial kits not conforming to proposed guidelines for these tests [11]. Such apparent inconsistencies limit clinical usefulness and effectiveness as well as interlaboratory comparability of LA, aCL, and anti-β_2GPI tests results. In general, aPL assays are very heterogeneous, poorly standardized, poorly harmonized, and consequently diversely sensitive and specific for APS. The standardization of autoantibodies assay is still a challenging task, and particularly limited progress has been made in the detection of aPL. Therefore, comparison studies are needed to further analyze the agreement between the different technologies.

It is well known that different assays for the detection of aPL show different sensitivities. By one plausible speculation LA assay is relatively "undersensitive" to aPL, so that only higher titre and more clinically relevant forms of aPL are detected by the clot-based tests [31]. On the other hand, immunoassays, such as aCL, may be "oversensitive," as they detect both clinically relevant and clinically irrelevant (e.g., infection-associated) forms of aPL. Furthermore, aCL test more often detect "low levels" of aPL that are less likely associated with APS than LA assay. The hypothesis is also supported by the observation that a positive result in the anti-β_2GPI assay (which is theoretically more "specific" but less "sensitive" than aCL for APS), is more strongly associated with clinical features of APS such as thrombosis than a positive result in the standard aCL assay [30]. For the physician, it is important to have in mind there is no gold standard aPL assay when defining the presence or absence of APS. However, data are emerging that the combination of multiple aPL findings is a superior risk stratification tool for clinical events in APS such as thrombosis [32, 33]. According to the revised classification criteria, APS patients should be divided into four categories: category I includes patients with more than one positive test in any combination, while patients with a single positive test should be classified in category II (IIa if LA positive, IIb if positive for antibodies against CL (aCLs), and IIc if positive for anti-β_2GPI antibodies) [11]. Triple positivity, defined by the presence of LA and medium/high titers of aCL and anti-β_2GPI antibodies (above the 99th percentile), is the most predictive profile for clinical manifestations and recurrences despite conventional treatment [34–36]. Patients in category II, expressing single aPL positivity, have a lesser risk to develop APS manifestations.

2.1. Lupus Anticoagulants (LA)

LA denotes a subgroup of aPL antibodies that prolong phospholipid-dependant clotting reactions. The clotting-based nature of the LA assay is fraught with preanalytical limitations, the need for multiple reagents, diversity in platforms, as well as challenges with interpreting results. It was shown that the presence of LA correlates better with thromboembolic complications than the presence of aCL [4]. The superiority of LA over aCL was explained by the nature of the assay; LA measures the activity of aPL, while in an ELISA, both the antibodies that influence functional activity and the antibodies that have no aPL activity are measured [37]. However, LA testing has several drawbacks, such as the absence of a reference method, low degree of standardization, and difficult test result interpretation. Consensus guidelines for the detection of LA were first published in the 1990s [38, 39]. Significant improvement in standardization has been achieved with the updated guidelines of the Scientific Standardization Subcommittee (SSC) of the International Society Thrombosis and Haemostasis in 2009 [40] and with the Clinical and Laboratory Standards Institute (CLSI) document in 2014 [41] that has resolved several issues of the preanalytical, analytical, and post-analytical phase.

The preanalytical phase plasma preparation is the crucial step. Plasma for LA analysis must be rendered platelet poor (platelet count less than 10×10^9/L), as residual platelets contain phospholipids that can shorten clotting times and generate false-negative results. Double centrifugation of blood is preferred, although a single centrifugation can also be suitable if the recommended platelet count is achieved. Ultracentrifugation as the second step is discouraged due to possible generation of phospholipid-containing microparticles [42]. Filtration through 0.22 μm cellulose acetate filters is also discouraged because of the binding of coagulation factors V, VIII, IX, XII, and von Willebrand factor to the filter [43]. Whether assays, such as dilute Russell's viper venom time (dRVVT), that bypass these coagulation factors are affected by filtration has not yet been studied.

Testing may be performed on fresh or properly frozen/thawed samples [41]. According to our experience, however, all the samples should be treated in the same manner as were plasma samples of healthy donors from which the reference values were obtained. For example, we found significantly longer activated partial thromboplastin times (APTTs) measured with the Staclot LA (Diagnostica Stago, France) on Behring Coagulation Timer (Dade Behring, Germany) in fresh (73.0 ± 17.7 s screening and 59.6 ± 12.1 s confirming test) compared to frozen/thawed plasma (59.8 ± 9.3 s screening and 53.7 ± 4.2 s confirming test, both paired t-test $p < 0.05$), while no differences were found for the dRVVT assay.

Several plasma-based (clotting) assays were traditionally used for LA detection that include intrinsic, extrinsic, or common coagulation pathway. On one hand, no single assay is 100% sensitive and specific for LA; therefore, the use of more than one assay was recommended. On the other hand, by increasing the number of different assays, the probability of false-positive results increases [44]. Guidelines therefore suggest using (no more than) two assays that are known to be responsive to LA, preferably dRVVT and APTT [41, 44].

Several strategies that include screening and confirming tests (with or without the mixing test) can be used for LA detection (Figure 2). In the screening test, low phospholipid levels are used, while confirmation test, preferably based on the same principle as the screening test, utilizes high phospholipid levels.

Each laboratory should establish its own cutoff value for a screening test above which confirming (and mixing) test needs to be performed. The SSC guidelines recommend using the 99th percentile [44], while the CLSI guidelines recommend average + 2 standard deviations (equal to 97.5th percentile) as the appropriate cutoff [41]. It should be noted that a higher cutoff insures less false-positive results, but a false-positive screening test from a statistical outlier in case of the lower cutoff will not generate false-positive composite interpretation. Yet a false-negative result in case of the higher cutoff could lead to inappropriate diagnosis and treatment [42].

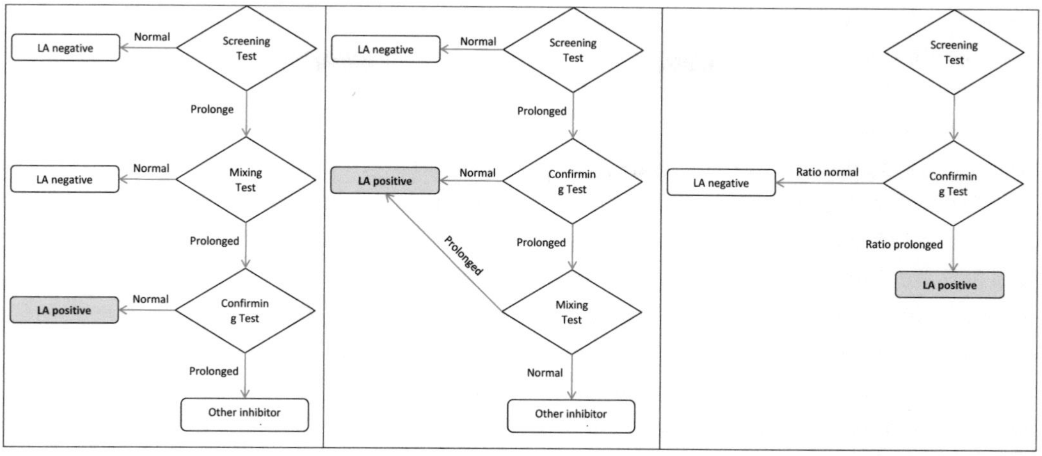

Figure 2. Strategies for LA detection. LA: lupus anticoagulant.

The need for a mixing test has been highly debated. When using an integrated test system (Figure 1, right panel), a mixing step is not necessary, and many laboratories avoid this step because of the additional work, cost, testing time, and the need for normal pool plasma. In addition, it is not clear how the mixing test should be performed (patient to normal pool plasma volume ratio, incubation time). Finally, there is some evidence that the mixing step produces false-negative results where a weak but clinically relevant LA is present [45]. On the other hand, integrated test systems without the mixing step may produce false-positive [46] as well as false-negative results [34]; therefore, further studies are needed.

LA testing results should be expressed as the normalized screen to confirm ratio [41, 44] as this practice reduces the variability of the analyzer and reagent performance. When the result is positive, additional assays, such as prothrombin time (to exclude vitamin K antagonists), thrombin time (to exclude heparin or direct thrombin inhibitor), and anti-Xa (to exclude low-molecular-weight heparin or direct factor Xa inhibitor), may be performed to make sure that the patient is not on anticoagulant therapy. The test panel should be repeated at or beyond 12 weeks to determine persistence of the LA [41, 44]. Laboratories should provide the final interpretation of LA testing results as positive (LA present), negative (LA not detected), or inconclusive (to be retested).

LA testing remains much more labor intensive and complicated to perform than ELISA but must be performed in parallel with aCL and anti-β_2GPI. Significant improvement has been achieved through SSC guidelines [44], but some issues are still unresolved and further reports of the SSC are awaited.

2.2. Anticardiolipin antibodies

The first molecularly defined aCL test was a radioimmunoassay established in 1983, using cardiolipin as an antigen, with a mixture of gelatin/PBS to dilute patient serum and radiolabeled anti-human IgG or IgM secondary antibodies. In 1990, three groups independently reported that aCL do not bind to cardiolipin in the absence of serum proteins, as summarized by Roubey [47]. The designation is somewhat misleading because aCL are an undefined group of antibodies that bind directly (1) to the cardiolipin (CL) and (2) to various (usually calf or bovine) serum proteins (most likely β_2GPI) linked to CL. The first group are β_2GPI-independent aCL (binding to CL does not require this cofactor), which are often associated with infectious diseases. Infectious aCL do not pose a risk for the occurrence of clinical signs associated with APS and are therefore indicated as nonthrombogenic autoantibodies. Infectious diseases can therefore determine the transient aCL positivity. Patients with syphilis, HIV, Lyme disease, and other infections triggered by cytomegalovirus, hepatitis C, and Epstein–Barr viruses may be mistakenly diagnosed as APS based on high levels of aCL especially, when concomitant arterial thrombosis or cerebrovascular accident is present [48]. In the second group, antibodies against β_2GPI prevail. These are the β_2GPI-dependent aCL antibodies (aCL/β_2GPI), which require the presence of cofactor β_2GPI for their binding to CL. They are characteristic of autoimmune diseases, as high titers of these antibodies detected in plasma represent a risk for thromboembolic complications. Therefore, for the detection of aCL (IgG and IgM), an ELISA method is used [49, 50], which measures the immune reactivity to CL as a phospholipid or to β_2GPI as a protein bound to phospholipids. The affinity of β_2GPI for CL is 30 to 40 times higher than affinity to phosphatidylserine [51]. Briefly, the ELISA test involves medium binding microtitre plates coated with highly purified negatively charged CL incubated overnight at 4°C and diluted patients sample in bovine serum (FBS), which acts as a cofactor for the recognition of CL as the antigen. After 2.5 h incubation at room temperature and two washes, goat antihuman IgG or IgM conjugated with alkaline phosphatase diluted in FBS/PBS was applied to the plates. Following washing, para-nitrophenylphosphate in diethanolamine buffer (pH 9.8) was applied, and optical density at 405 nm (OD405) was kinetically measured by a spectrometer (Figure 3) [50, 52]. The essential weakness of this assay is that patients with aCL antibodies that bind human but not bovine β_2GPI can be missed. Therefore, some laboratories use human β_2GPI instead of bovine or calf serum as a source of β_2GPI in the aCL ELISA.

Several international workshops and forums have been conducted in an attempt to standardize the aCL test [53–58]. Despite these efforts, a considerable degree of interlaboratory variation still exists [59]. There is also a high degree of variability between different commercial kits for the detection of aCL even when assessed within the same laboratory, with lower variability seen with different commercial anti-β_2GPI kits [60]. This keeps raising the question of the standardization of commercial and/or in-house laboratory methods and results [61]. Although laboratory results represent an essential contribution to the diagnosis of APS, many questions regarding methodology and reference values of various in-house and commercially available kits that are not comparable still remain unanswered. In an effort to improve the diagnostic value of aPL antibody assays, aCL determination is still necessary and should be complemented by anti-β_2GPI determination in accordance with revised Sydney laboratory classification criteria for the diagnosis of APS [11].

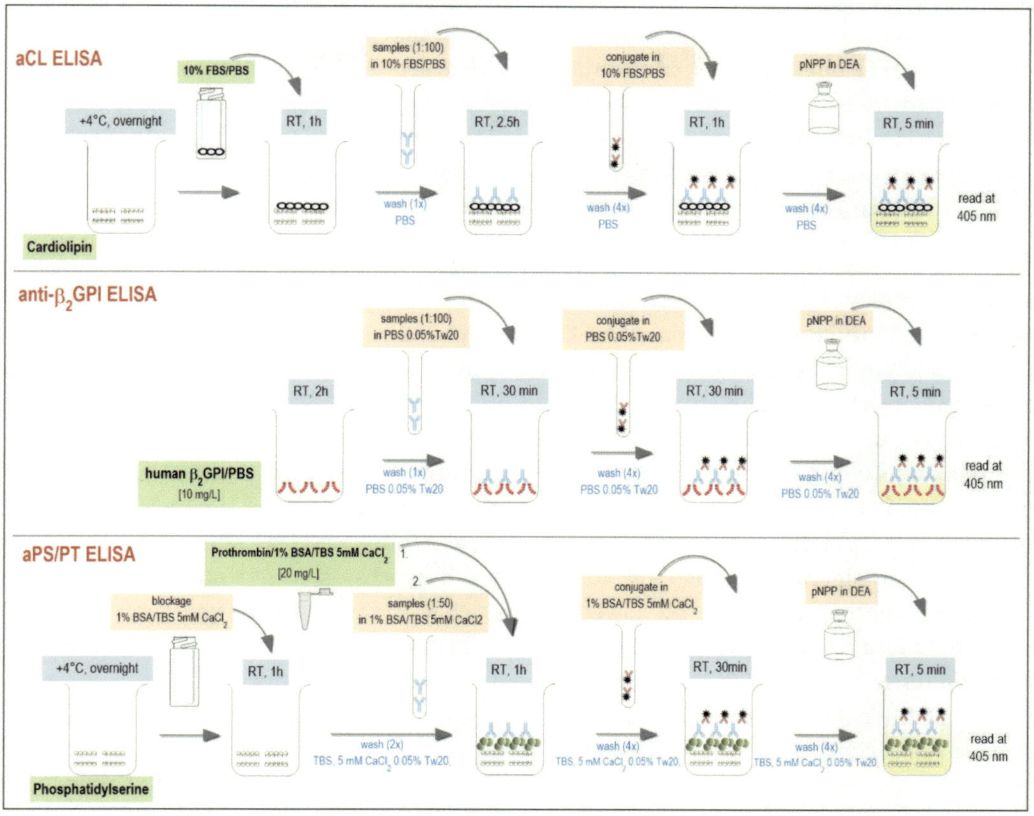

Figure 3. Laboratory protocols for aCL, anti-β_2GPI, and aPS/PT ELISA. BSA: bovine serum albumin; conjugate: goat antihuman IgG/M/A conjugated with alkaline phosphatase; DEA: diethanolamine buffer; FBS: fetal bovine serum; PBS: phosphate-buffered saline; pNPP: para-nitrophenylphosphate; RT: room temperature; TBS: tris buffer saline; Tw20: Tween-20.

2.3. Antibodies against β_2GPI

A large part of autoantibodies in patients with APS are directed against β_2GPI and anti-β_2GPI therefore represent one of the main subgroups of antiphospholipid antibodies [62]. β_2GPI, also known as apolipoprotein H, is a multifunctional and evolutionary conserved single-chain glycosylated protein present in plasma at concentrations ~180 mg/L (range 20–300 mg/L) [63–65]. The major site of β_2GPI synthesis is the liver, although its mRNA has also been found in endothelial cells, neurons, astrocytes, and in the extra villous cytotrophoblast and syncytio-trophoblast of placenta [66]. The ~50-kDa protein consists of 326 amino acids, which are folded into five short consensus repeat domains, termed also "sushi" domains. Domains I–IV are composed of ~ 60 amino acids, and each contains two disulfide bridges, while the domain V consists of 82 amino acids. Domain V also has specific characteristics, such as a positively charged, lysine-rich region, a hydrophobic loop, and a 19-residue C-terminal extension, which is cross-linked by an additional disulfide bond allowing β_2GPI to bind to negatively charged phospholipids [67–70]. Due to specific interactions between the domains I and V of β_2GPI, the protein exists in three configurations, i.e., circular plasma protein, as observed by electronic microscopy [71], open fishhook conformation, as revealed by its crystal structure [69, 72], and an intermediate S-shape, which has been recently observed using small-angle X-ray scattering [73]. After binding to suitable anionic surface, for example, to phospholipids, β_2GPI changes its conformation from circular to open ("J"), exposing a cryptic epitope, which is recognized by anti-β_2GPI-directed against domain I [74].

Although routine laboratories detect and interpret anti-β_2GPI as one set of autoantibodies, they actually represent a very heterogeneous group directed against the same antigen. Due to their polyclonal nature subpopulations of anti-β_2GPI vary in epitope recognition [63, 75–78], avidity [79–82], and pathological mechanisms of their action [63, 83, 84], which results in their different pathogenicity and clinical relevance [63, 77, 78, 80, 85, 86]. A subset of IgG anti-β_2GPI directed against domain I on β_2GPI seems to have a prominent role in the pathology of thrombotic complications in patients with APS [74]. According to de Laat *et al.* [87], pathologic anti-β_2GPI can be divided into those targeting epitope on domain I (directed against the G40-R43 residues), which highly correlate with thrombosis, and those targeting nondomain I epitopes. According to Giannakopoulos *et al.* [88], these differences are due to anti-β_2GPI avidity. Therefore, avidity must also be considered when describing the diversity of anti-β_2GPI subpopulations and their clinical relevance. Several research groups/clinical studies indicated that difference in strength of binding to the same antigen/same epitope could be an important marker of the pathogenicity of the specific anti-β_2GPI subgroups [80, 85, 89]. An association between high-avidity IgG anti-β_2GPI and thrombotic or obstetric complications in patients with APS was reported [85, 90]. This was in contrast to low-avidity IgG anti-β_2GPI, which was more prevalent in autoimmune patients without APS. The involvement of high avidity IgG anti-β_2GPI in the pathogenesis of APS was also confirmed in an *in vitro* study on human coronary artery endothelial cells [91]. In this study, high-avidity IgG anti-β_2GPI was shown to increase the expression of inflammatory and chemotactic cytokines leading to higher migration of monocytes. These effects were further intensified in presence of the major acute phase protein serum amyloid A (SAA) [91], denoting that along with lipopolysaccharide [83], SAA as a marker of inflammation, also represents a trigger or a second hit uncovering the full pathological potential of anti-β_2GPI [91]. The differences among antigen binding sites on anti-β_2GPI of differently avidity were further confirmed by the location of the recognized epitopes on β_2GPI. Therefore, using heptamer phage display libraries two binding epitopes of high-avidity IgG anti-β_2GPI have been characterized: FNPYWYV and QGOAHSK [92]. These sequences mimicked specific amino acid clusters on domains II and III of β_2GPI and were accessible to high-avidity IgG anti-β_2GPI in the fishhook and circular conformations. In contrast, the sequence KMDGNHP has been characterized as a surface binding epitope for low-avidity IgG anti-β_2GPI located between domains III and IV of β_2GPI. It was accessible for the binding of low-avidity IgG anti-β_2GPI only in the open/fishhook conformation [92]. Epitopes of low-avidity IgG anti-β_2GPI are cryptic and not reachable for the antibodies when β_2GPI molecules occupy the closed plasma conformation, which explains a negligible binding of the respective anti-β_2GPI to β_2GPI in the solution. Epitopes of high-avidity IgG anti-β_2GPI are native and reachable regardless of conformation of the β_2GPI, which is in accordance with the proven binding of the respective anti-β_2GPI to antigen in the solution. High-avidity monoclonal anti-β_2GPI recognizes β_2GPI in the solution by binding to the epitope, which is crucial for the restoration of the closed conformation of the β_2GPI [81]. Since enzyme-linked immunosorbent assays currently used in routine diagnostics detect anti-β_2GPI antibodies of unknown avidity, these observations are potentially useful for the development of improved diagnostic tests capable of detecting clinically relevant antibodies. The avidity of IgG anti-β_2GPI was determined by chaotropic anti-β_2GPI ELISA [79]. The procedure was in principle the same as in the anti-β_2GPI ELISA, using chaotropic conditions during antibody binding. Samples were diluted in PBS–Tween containing increasing concentration of NaCl. Discrimination between anti-β_2GPI with high or low avidity was made arbitrarily, comparing the initial binding at 0.15 M NaCl with bindings at higher salt concentrations [79, 85]. NaCl (0.5 M) was selected as the reference concentration for comparison with the initial binding. When the binding at 0.5 M NaCl remained higher than 70% of the initial one, the presence of high-avidity anti-β_2GPI was declared. When the binding at 0.5 M NaCl decreased to or below 25% of the initial binding, low-avidity anti-β_2GPI were designated. Samples that did not fulfill either of the above criteria were considered to be of heterogeneous avidity [79].

The addition of anti-β_2GPI antibodies to the revised Sydney laboratory classification criteria for the diagnosis of APS was finalized in 2006 [11]. According to the consensus guidelines on anti-β_2GPI testing and reporting [93], IgG anti-β_2GPI should be performed on all requests for anti-β_2GPI where isotype is not specified. If both IgG and IgM anti-β_2GPI antibody testing is routinely performed on all requests (regardless of whether IgM anti-β_2GPI testing has been specifically requested), then it has been suggested that a comment should be provided to the physician indicating that the association between isolated positive IgM anti-β_2GPI results and thrombosis is uncertain but appears to be lower than for IgG anti-β_2GPI [93].

ELISA that measures the immune reactivity directly to β_2GPI is used for the detection of anti-β_2GPI (IgG and IgM). The characteristics are similar to the detection of aCL with the major difference that in anti-β_2GPI ELISA, the purified human native β_2GPI [94] is coated directly onto the ELISA microtitre plates. Briefly, high binding polystyrene microtitre plates were coated with β_2GPI in PBS and incubated with sera diluted in PBS containing 0.05% Tween-20. The detection system was the same as in aCL ELISA (Figure 3). Anti-β_2GPI is directed against a cryptic epitope exposed when β_2GPI is bound to anionic phospholipid or another suitable surface [95]. Namely, some brands of ELISA plates are unable to induce the conformational change due to difference in structure or charge and are unsuitable for use in anti-β_2GPI ELISA [95]. There remains a lack of a formal, universally accepted method for performing anti-β_2GPI ELISA, coupled with a lack of standardized WHO accepted calibrators. The in-house and commercial kits are calibrated by their own "calibrators" and expressed in arbitrary units. Consequently, there is a great variability in the results reported by the different laboratories. Meroni *et al.* suggested that the identification of common calibrators may be useful in obtaining more reproducible results [96]. Both polyclonal IgG/IgM anti-β_2GPI antibodies affinity-purified from two APS patients with high IgG and IgM anti-β_2GPI levels and chimeric monoclonal IgG antibody (INOVA, San Diego, CA, USA) reacting with human β_2GPI have been selected as candidates for reference material for calibration [97]. This reference material may contribute significantly to better standardization of anti-β_2GPI immunoassays.

3. Noncriteria aPL

The majority of APS patients have APS, as defined by the presence of clinical features and positive one or more laboratory criteria aPL. However, a small proportion of patients have significant clinical features of APS but lacking persistently elevated above-mentioned criteria aPL. These so-called "seronegative" APS patients (SNAPS) probably do exhibit certain aPL, which may not be identifiable given the limitations of currently available aPL assays. Even if such a patient does not fully satisfy the classification criteria, he/she may still have APS. Missing a diagnosis of APS in these individuals may lead to the absence of appropriate therapy and potentially significant adverse outcomes for such patients. For clinical studies, patients falling into any of these categories should be classified separately from those that fulfill the revised classification criteria for APS.

3.1. IgA aCL and IgA anti-β_2GPI antibodies

Although standard serological tests included in the current laboratory classification criteria for APS [11] detect IgG and IgM isotypes for the aCL and anti-β_2GPI but not the IgA isotype, clinicians will occasionally encounter patients with isolated IgA aPL who exhibit clinical manifestations of APS. Most studies to date have mainly focused on the IgG/IgM isotypes of aPL, with only rare reports pointing to the possible clinical significance of IgA aPL. The literature on IgA aPL is quite heterogeneous, reporting a high variability in their prevalence and clinical significance due to different study designs and populations studied and different laboratory methods (in-house as well as commercial kits) with different cutoffs and different ethnic populations (review in [98]). IgA aCL and anti-β_2GPI antibodies have been reported in up to 70% of patients with systemic lupus erythematosus (SLE) and in those with primary APS [98]. The role of IgA isotypes of both antibodies in APS is however unclear. Lagos *et al.* [99] found that livedo reticularis, heart valve disease, thrombocytopenia, and epilepsy are more common among subjects with increased IgA anti-β_2GPI antibodies [99]. A similar association was observed in SLE patients [100].

The reports on the prevalence of IgA aCL are extremely variable ranging from 0% to nearly 50% [28]. Altogether, twelve studies showed an association between IgA aCL and certain clinical features related to APS but fifteen studies failed to find any relationship between the presence of IgA aCL and the clinical signs of APS (review in [28]). Studies investigating diagnostic applicability and added value of IgA aCL determination show a general weakness, seeing as elevated value of IgA aCL are often accompanied with positive IgG and/or IgM aCL, making it difficult to understand the role of elevated IgA aCL alone. In addition, a great variability of results suggests that studies are barely comparable in the population included, regarding methods used and results obtained. Some differences among studies can also be due to different ethnicity. IgA seems to be the most prevalent isotype of aCL in African Americans [101], African Caribbean [102], and Japanese patients [103].

There is also a controversy in the literature regarding the meaning of elevated IgA anti-β_2GPI. The majority of published papers have highlighted the value of IgA anti-β_2GPI in the diagnosis of APS [28]. Thrombosis, particularly arterial thrombosis [86, 104, 105], is frequently found associated with IgA anti-β_2GPI, although the simultaneous presence of other isotypes makes it often difficult to interpret. Mehrani *et al.* [106] reported on a high prevalence of IgA aPL antibodies with 20% positive IgA anti-β_2GPI associated with deep vein thrombosis. IgA anti-β_2GPI seems to be more prevalent in SLE patients compared to IgA aCL (review in [98]). Therefore, IgA anti-β_2GPI have gained clinical relevance and were recently included among aPL tests in the novel SLICC classification criteria for SLE [107]. Ruiz-García *et al.* [108] also suggested that the assessment of IgA anti-β_2GPI in patients with suspected primary APS is important for the identification, treatment, and management of patients who in accordance with the current classification criteria are not diagnosed at this point of the disease since the serological profile of patients with primary APS (where IgA is the most prevalent isotype) is different from systemic autoimmune disorders-associated APS (where IgG is the most prevalent isotype). Therefore, in selected patients where the clinical suspicion of APS is high but all tests for other antiphospholipid antibodies are negative, testing for IgA anti-β_2GPI might be clinically useful and therefore recommended [58, 93, 109]. Despierres *et al.* [105] also proposed that IgA anti-β_2GPI should be searched for in all patients with unexplained thrombosis based on their finding that IgA anti-β_2GPI was associated with thrombosis even in non-SLE patients. Most patients positive for IgA anti-β_2GPI were negative for IgA aCL [108, 109].

In addition, a subpopulation of IgA anti-β_2GPI directed against domain IV has been linked to atherosclerosis in a study using different β_2GPI domain-deleted mutants and native β_2GPI [86]. Akhter *et al.* also reported that in a large cohort of nearly 300 SLE patients, the only assay with a significant association with stroke was the IgA anti-β_2GPI directed against domain IV/V [104].

3.2. Anti-domain I β_2GPI antibodies

For better clinical diagnosis and management of APS, a lot of efforts have been implicated for better characterization of pathogenic function and clinical significance of anti-β_2GPI. Several groups have studied the fine specificity of anti-β_2GPI, and every domain of β_2GPI has been described to bind antibodies [63]. From an immunologic point of view, it is hard to imagine a self-protein containing many immunodominant epitopes. Therefore, many studies have been initiated to identify the most immunodominant epitope. Most evidence points to the domain I (DI) of β_2GPI. A specific epitope in DI is a positively charged discontinuous structure located in the N-terminal of β_2GPI and has been identified as the most relevant antigenic target involved in the binding of anti-β_2GPI to β_2GPI [110]. The reactivity to DI was first described by Iverson *et al.* in 1998, who showed that most anti-β_2GPI reacted with DI of β_2GPI using domain-deletion mutants of the protein [111]. The binding of anti-DI anti-β_2GPI (anti-β_2GPI-DI) to β_2GPI is conformation dependent [110]. In the circular conformation of β_2GPI, DI interacts with domain V, and immunodominant epitope is therefore hidden. When β_2GPI takes the intermediate S-shape, the epitope in the DI is covered by carbohydrate chains of domain III and domain IV, thus preventing the binding of antibodies to β_2GPI [74]. The binding of β_2GPI to the anionic surface may induce conformational change of β_2GPI from circular to J-shaped conformation, which also results in the displacement of the domains III–IV carbohydrate side chains; the critical epitope arginine 39-glycine 43 is exposed and thus becomes accessible for domain-specific anti-β_2GPI binding [74]. Despite a wide interest in the potential diagnostic value of these DI-specific antibodies in the diagnosis of APS, specifically anti-β_2GPI-DI, the number of studies is still limited, and their potential clinical utility has not been widely accepted [112]. Anti-β_2GPI-DI antibodies have attracted particular interest as they are strongly associated with thrombosis [77, 113–115]. Ciesla *et al.* [116] found that increased IgG anti-β_2GPI-DI antibodies were associated with livedo reticularis and heart valve disease in APS, which is also in concordance with the finding of de Laat and coworkers [63]. The later have also reported of IgG anti-β_2GPI-DI antibodies to be associated with heart valve disease presumably linked to thrombotic processes on a valve with autoimmune valvulitis, being a risk factor for stroke.

To date, there have been no commercial kits to detect anti-β_2GPI-DI antibodies available on the market; however, several research methods have been developed [110]. As the binding of anti-β_2GPI-DI antibodies might be directly affected with conformational changes of β_2GPI, the preparation and coating β_2GPI to ELISA trays is of major importance for the results of the assay. It has been consistently observed that anti-β_2GPI-DI antibodies react with their target epitope only when DI is bound onto hydrophobic but not hydrophilic surface. The majority of studies used the two steps ELISA using β_2GPI-DI coated on hydrophobic and hydrophilic microtitre plates [110, 113, 117]. This method is based on the assumption that the epitope of β_2GPI-DI is exposed only to the hydrophilic surface of the microtitre plates and thus accessible for autoantibody binding [113]. Pozzi *et al.* showed that the capture ELISA with chemical synthesized N-terminally biotinylated β_2GPI-DI on streptavidin plates was able to discriminate between APS patients and controls in contrast to nonbiotinylated β_2GPI-DI directly immobilized onto ELISA plates [118]. A liquid phase inhibition assay using a whole β_2GPI immobilized on the solid phase and synthetic β_2GPI-DI as inhibitor was also developed [119]. In addition, Iverson and coworkers developed an ELISA, which was based on recombinant β_2GPI-DI expressed and purified from insect cells [120]. Recently, a novel β_2GPI-DI chemiluminescence immunoassay (CIA, INOVA Diagnostics, San Diego, USA) based on the BIO-FLASH system (Biokit, Barcelona, Spain) and using a recombinant β_2GPI-DI coupled to paramagnetic beads has been developed [121]. Despite comparability between solid phase assays and a CIA immunoassay, results obtained by both approaches should be evaluated in a larger multicentre studies in order to confirm the reproducibility of different anti-β_2GPI-DI antibody assays. It is also premature to replace the anti-β_2GPI ELISA with the anti-β_2GPI-DI assays, as there is still the possibility that other populations of thrombosis related antibodies are present.

3.3. Antiprothrombin antibodies

Prothrombin, a phospholipid binding protein, was first proposed as a possible co-factor for LA by Loeliger in 1959 [122]. In 1983, Bajaj and his colleagues were the first to ascertain the evidence of prothrombin binding antibodies in two patients with LA and severe hypoprothrombinemia [123]. These antibodies bound prothrombin without preventing its activation to thrombin. The authors assumed that the hypoprothrombinemia resulted in a rapid removal of prothrombin–antibody complexes from circulation. A year later, the existence of prothrombin–antiprothrombin immune complex was confirmed with counterimmunoelectrophoresis (CIE) in the plasma of patients with LA, but without hypoprothrombinemia [124]. Fleck *et al.*

http://dx.doi.org/10.5772/61551

confirmed these findings, showing that 74% of patients with LA had evidence of anti-prothrombin antibodies on CIE and that antiprothrombin antibodies exhibit LA activity [125]. Bevers *et al.* highlighted the role of antiprothrombin antibodies for the LA activity in patients with elevated aCL and LA [126]. In eleven out of sixteen patients' sera, the binding to phospholipid surface was detected only in the presence of prothrombin and calcium ions. Later, Oosting and his colleagues demonstrated that antibodies with LA activity inhibited prothrombinase complexes on the surface of endothelial cells and that IgG fraction with LA activity bound the phospholipid-prothrombin immune complexes [127]. A review elucidated that majority of antibodies with LA activity bind prothrombin and/or β_2GPI [128]. Double diffusion and CIE were the first techniques used for the detection of antiprothrombin antibodies [123–125, 129]. Their main advantage was in the measurement of prothrombin–antiprothrombin immune complexes. These *in vitro* findings have indicated that such complexes might exist in plasma, but detection methods used did not enable quantitative measurements. In many cases, the titer and/or affinity of antiprothrombin antibodies were too low to obtain a clear precipitation line. Other techniques based their detection on the impairment of enzyme activity of prothrombin after binding with relevant antibodies [127, 130]. The need for isolation of antiprothrombin antibodies and purification of clotting factors makes these methods unsuitable for routine work.

In the last few years, several research groups developed various ELISAs, which are by far most widely used techniques for the determination of antiprothrombin antibodies, since they enable relatively quick determination of a titre and antibody isotype. Arvieux *et al.* first presented an ELISA, where prothrombin as the antigen was applied to high binding microtitre plates [131]. In this way, they determined antibodies directed against prothrombin alone (aPT-A or aPT). It is important to note that the manner of prothrombin presentation on a solid surface greatly affects its recognition by antiprothrombin antibodies [132]. Antiprothrombin antibodies only bind prothrombin when immobilized on an appropriate anionic surface such as γ-irradiated or high binding polyvinylchloride (PVC) microtitre plates, or to prothrombin exposed to the immobilized anionic phospholipids. Antiprothrombin antibodies cannot be detected when prothrombin is immobilized on nonirradiated plates [131]. In this respect, the reactivity of antiprothrombin antibodies in an ELISA strongly resembles the reactivity of low-avidity anti-β_2GPI. The latter recognizes β_2GPI only when bound to the anionic surface, while their binding to the antigen in liquid phase is minimal [133–135]. Matsuuda *et al.* [136] showed that antiprothrombin antibodies could be detected also by an ELISA where prothrombin is bound to immobilized phosphatidylserine (aPS/PT ELISA). Soon it was shown that aPS/PT ELISA was more efficient in determination of antiprothrombin antibodies in comparison to aPT ELISA [137]. The phenomenon can be explained in several ways: (1) prothrombin, bound to phosphatidylserine, is not limited in its lateral movement, in contrast with prothrombin bound to high-binding microtitre plates resulting in clustering and proper orientation of prothrombin offering better conditions for antibody binding; (2) ELISA with phosphatidylserine in solid phase may, through the calcium ions, capture the circulating prothrombin–antiprothrombin immune complexes present in certain samples; and (3) antiprothrombin antibodies may react with neoepitopes occurring on prothrombin molecules only when bound to phosphatidylserine through calcium ions. Altogether, aPS/PT ELISA better simulates the *in vivo* conditions, where prothrombin and antiprothrombin antibodies presumably bind to phospholipid surface of endothelial cells. In addition, Atsumi *et al.* showed that the aPS/PT strongly correlated with LA activity [138]. This group showed there was no correlation between the levels of aPS/PT and aPT in patients with APS and therefore assumed that the aPS/PT ELISA determines, at least in part, different antibodies compared to aPT ELISA. The first published aPS/PT protocol was later modified in order to increase the analytical sensitivity of the test [139]. The modified procedure allowed the detection of the two allegedly different populations of antibodies and thus determination of all clinically relevant antiprothrombin antibodies with one method. The authors reported that their in-house aPS/PT ELISA was the most optimal method for the determination of all clinically relevant aPS/PT antibodies, exhibiting the highest percentage of LA activity, compared to aCL and anti-β_2GPI [139]. The ELISA protocol is schematically presented in Figure 3. Briefly, medium binding plates were coated with phosphatidylserine in chloroform/methanol 1:4 and dried overnight at 4°C. Following blocking with Tris-buffered saline (TBS) containing 1% bovine serum albumin (BSA) and 5 mM $CaCl_2$ (1% BSA/TBS-Ca) and two washes with 5 mM $CaCl_2$-TBS–0.05% Tween 20 (TBS-Tw), human prothrombin of final concentration 10 mg/L and patients' sera diluted 1:100 were applied to wells immediately one after the other and incubated for 1 h at room temperature. After 4 washes, alkaline-conjugated goat anti-human IgG or IgM were applied in 1% BSA/TBS-Ca and incubated for 30 min. Following 4 washes in TBS/Tw, 100 μl/well of para-nitrophenylphosphate in diethanolamine buffer (pH 9.8) was applied and OD405 was kinetically measured by a spectrometer (Figure 3). Zigon *et al.* also showed that antiprothrombin antibodies are of different avidity, which greatly impacts their detection by different ELISAs [139, 140]. It was shown that low-avidity antiprothrombin antibodies were detectable only in the aPS/PT ELISA, while aPT ELISA detected only antibodies with predominantly heterogeneous avidity. Initially, only a few commercial kits for the detection of antiprothrombin antibodies were available, and they all measured aPT antibodies. Their overall diagnostic sensitivity and specificity was poor [141]. In 2010, the commercial QUANTA Lite™ aPS/PT IgG/IgM and LAC assays became available as an aid to the diagnosis of APS [15, 142]. Zigon *et al.* showed that results measured with QUANTA Lite™ aPS/PT highly correlated with their modified in-house procedure described above and confirmed that both ELISAs have high diagnostic specificity and sensitivity for APS [15].

Several retrospective and cross-sectional studies, which were first summarized in Galli *et al.* [143] and recently in Sciasca *et al.* [14], had examined the clinical significance of antibodies to prothrombin determined by ELISA. Different laboratories performed their variation of ELISA methods using commercially available assay kits for the determination of antibodies to prothrombin. International studies that have attempted to standardize and unify these methods were very rare [141]. The main reasons for significant differences in results among published studies are modified procedures, different reagents used, and the fact that international standards are not available. Comparative studies of two methods aPT or aPS/PT ELISA showed that the results only partially overlap, which means that some patients were positive in only one ELISA [141, 144–146]. Researchers then speculated that results from aPT ELISA and from aPS/PT ELISA allegedly do not belong to the same population of antibodies, although both are clinically associated with APS. Many have therefore estimated that in terms of clinical significance, it is necessary to consider the results of the two performances. A recent systematic review of studies on aPT (38 studies) and aPS/PT (10 studies) summarizes the results of more than 7000 patients and controls. Both types of antiprothrombin antibodies represent an increased risk for thrombosis, but meta-analysis in the article showed that elevated aPS/PT pose a greater risk for

http://dx.doi.org/10.5772/61551

arterial and/or venous thrombosis compared with aPT (OR = 5.1, 95% CI = 4.2 to 6.3 and OR = 1.8, 95% CI = 1.4 to 2.8). The authors concluded that routine measurements of aPS/PT, but not aPT, allow better insight to thrombotic risk in patients with systemic autoimmune diseases as well as confirm an undeniable need for further research toward the inclusion of these antibodies in laboratory criteria for APS.

Results of a modified aPS/PT ELISA [15] have shown that elevated aPS/PT represent an increased risk of venous thrombosis (OR = 3.5, 95% CI = 1.7 to 7.0) and less so for arterial thrombosis (OR = 1.9, 95% CI = 0.9 to 4.1) (Table 1). A very important finding was that antibodies to prothrombin compared to other aPL (LA, aCL, and anti-β_2GPI) represented the highest risk for pregnancy complications (OR = 9.3, 95% CI = 3.5 to 24.6). Not many studies have investigated the relationship between antibodies to prothrombin and complications during pregnancy, and about half of these studies have not confirmed such correlations [145, 147–150]. In contrast, Akimoto [151] and Bertolaccini [152] and their colleagues showed strong and specific association between different types of antibodies to prothrombin and miscarriages. Clinical correlations between antibodies and late pregnancy complications were later confirmed by two other studies [153, 154], but none of the studies found any link between complications in early pregnancy before 12 weeks of pregnancy and the presence of antibodies to prothrombin. The most recent study clearly showed an overall prevalence of aPS/PT of 13.0%, aCL of 12.4%, LA, and anti-β_2GPI less than 8.0% in a group of patients with obstetric complications characteristic for APS. Both aPS/PT and aCL were significantly more prevalent compared to healthy blood donors. However, aCL correlated only with late pregnancy morbidity and prematurity, while aPS/PT were the only antibodies associated with early recurrent pregnancy loss, as well as with late pregnancy morbidity and prematurity. Authors suggested that, aPS/PT measurement might improve the evaluation of patients with early recurrent pregnancy loss, undiscovered by other aPL tests [155].

		Arterial thrombosis (n=41)				*Venous thrombosis (n=53)*				*Obstetric complications (n=28)*			
Antibody		*p-value*	*Odds ratio (95% CI)*	*Sensitivity %*	*Specificity %*	*p-value*	*Odds ratio (95% CI)*	*Sensitivity %*	*Specificity %*	*p-value*	*Odds ratio (95% CI)*	*Sensitivity %*	*Specificity %*
LA		0.43	1.4 (0.6-2.9)	49	59	<0.001	5.6 (2.6-12.2)	70	70	<0.005	4.3 (1.6-11.9)	62	73
aCL	IgG	<0.001	5.5 (2.3-13.4)	83	53	<0.005	3.0 (1.5-6.2)	74	52	<0.001	5.8 (2.1-15.9)	79	61
	IgM	0.67	1.2 (0.4-3.5)	15	88	0.010	3.5 (1.3-9.2)	23	92	0.130	2.5 (0.8-7.8)	21	90
anti-β_2GPI	IgG	0.02	2.4 (1.2-5.1)	63	58	<0.001	3.2 (1.6-6.5)	66	63	0.002	4.1 (1.7-10.4)	68	66
	IgM	0.99	1.0 (0.3-2.9)	12	88	0.070	2.5 (0.9-6.5)	19	91	0.278	2.0 (0.6-6.6)	18	90
aPS/PT	IgG	0.08	1.9 (0.9-4.1	44	71	<0.001	3.5 (1.7-7.0)	51	77	<0.001	9.3 (3.5-24.6)	64	84
	IgM	0.36	1.4 (0.6-2.9)	39	69	0.021	2.2 (1.1-4.5)	45	73	<0.005	4.0 (1.6-9.9)	54	78

Table 1. Antiphospholipid antibodies and LA in relationship to arterial thrombosis (AT), venous thrombosis (VT), and obstetric complications (OC). aCL: anticardiolipin; anti-β_2GPI: anti-$\beta_2$glycoprotein; aPS/PT anti-phosphatidylserine/prothrombin; LA: lupus anticoagulant; OR: odds ratio; CI: confidence interval.

4. Novel/future methodology

Given the poor standardization of single aPL testing, new technical approaches to aPL profiling have been proposed recently, which elucidated the possibility of aPL profiling for the diagnosis of APS and outcome prediction [22, 24, 156]. In order to ensure the quality of routine laboratory measurements, along with time and cost-efficiency, multiline immunodot assays or bead-based multiplex techniques might represent a solution for these challenges. Apart from the immunodot technique, the detection of aPL by flow cytometry using beads with particular surface properties seems to represent another promising approach in aPL antibody multiplex testing [23]. In the future, we can also expect studies exploring miRNAs as biomarkers for risk of thrombosis and/or obstetric complication. Many miRNAs have been found significantly altered in sera or plasma of patients with thrombosis [25] or specific pregnancy complications [26, 27].

4.1. Multiplex assays

Recently, the parallel detection of aCL and anti-β_2GPI antibodies of IgG, IgA, and IgM isotypes related to APS was developed in the BioPlex system (BioPlex™ 2200 multiplex immunoassay system using APLS reagents). A unique fully automated multiplex immunoassay platform that allows the qualitative and quantitative measurements of several antibodies was developed [24]. The instrument combines the multianalyte profiling technology with antigen-coated fluoromagnetic beads as the solid phase, in an automated platform where sampling, processing, and data reduction are performed automatically. Unlike other methods, beads are washed after incubation and labeling; magnetic beads are used to automate washing steps and support random access testing [157]. The BioPlex APLS system seems to have a good diagnostic accuracy for all tests. However, the simultaneous detection of aCL and anti-β_2GPI of IgA isotype together with IgG and IgM isotypes did not increase the diagnostic sensitivity for APS. This was the first and until now the only study on the BioPlex APLS system; therefore, the applicability of this technology needs to be further explored and confirmed.

4.2. Multiline immunodot assays

A multiline immunodot assay (MLDA) uses a different solid phase and is an alternative to ELISA for simultaneous assessment of multiple aPL. Only one research group reported the use of hydrophobic membrane as the solid phase for immobilization of phospholipids in aPL antibody testing [22, 156, 158, 159]. The anionic phospholipids CL, phosphatidylinositol, and phosphatidylserine were immobilized in lines together with the co-factor protein β_2GPI and a reaction control reactant on a polyvinylidene difluoride (PVDF) membrane strip to detect specific autoantibodies simultaneously in one sample. Membrane surfaces like the hydrophobic PVDF membrane seemed to induce surprisingly the same conformational changes in the β_2GPI polypeptide required for disease-specific aPL. It may be assumed that the membrane immobilization mimics the *in vivo* presentation of anionic phospholipids in membranes more appropriately since the majority of aPL antibodies are supposed to be of medium or rather low affinity and bivalent binding is required for strong amplification of interaction. The formation of multiple interconnected immune complexes on an appropriate lipid surface might be of importance for antibody testing. Authors of the study explained that MLDA provided the appropriate reaction environment for the detection of three different aPL antibody reactivities. First, aPL antibodies to pure anionic phospholipids were determined; second, immobilized

http://dx.doi.org/10.5772/61551

phospholipids interacting with cofactor-aPL antibody complexes were detected; and third, antibodies against cofactor proteins alone could be detected. Therefore, this technique may assess a broader spectrum of reactivity in a multiplex format for aPL antibody profiling than the recommended ELISA technique does. However, the inability of quantification and the lack of confirmation by other researchers make this very novel methodology questionable.

4.3. miRNAs

MicroRNAs (miRNAs) are small noncoding RNAs with 21 to 25 nucleotides in length that posttranslationally regulate gene expression. miRNAs are fundamentally involved in the regulation of major biological processes in health and disease. The primary miRNA sequence repository—miRBase database (http://www.mirbase.org/), the latest miRBase release (v20, June 2013), contains 24521 miRNA loci from 206 species, processed to produce 30424 mature miRNA products [160].

Since the discovery that miRNAs are highly stable in circulation [161, 162], circulating serum/ plasma miRNAs have gained an extensive research interest as highly promising noninvasive clinical biomarkers in diagnosis, prognosis, treatment response, and risk assessment in several diseases, including cancer [163, 164] autoimmune diseases [165, 166], myocardial infarction [167], heart failure [168], deep vein thrombosis [169], and pregnancy complications (reviewed in [170, 171]).

Williams *et al.* showed that the vast majority of circulating miRNAs in healthy human plasma originated from blood components and endothelial cells, and tissue-specific miRNAs from gut and liver were represented as well [172]. This suggested broad tissue contribution to the circulating pool of miRNAs in healthy human plasma. In contrast, skeletal muscle-, heart-, and brain-specific miRNAs were detected only at very low levels in healthy plasma, suggesting that such miRNAs, when detected in circulation at increased levels may specifically reflect source tissue damage or disease. The strong evidence for the existence of the circulating organ-specific miRNAs in tissue damage or disease comes, for example, from the study of circulating miRNAs in myocardial injury in patients with advanced heart failure [168]. In this study, cardiac-specific (miR-208b, miR-208a, and miR-449) and muscle-specific (miR-1-1 and miR-133b) circulating miRNAs (myomirs) increased up to 140-fold in patients with advanced heart failure as compared to subject without heart disease and highly correlated to the levels of cardiac troponin I, the established marker of heart injury.

The potential for shedding the tissue-specific miRNAs in the circulation during organ damage or disease, alongside their high stability in serum and plasma, equips circulating tissue-specific miRNAs with high potential for clinical biomarker applications. However, to reach significant levels in the circulation, tissue-specific miRNA biomarker has to be abundantly present in the damaged source tissue as, for example, in advanced heart failure [168]. In addition, the source tissue has to be well perfused and of considerable size to be able to contribute to the circulating miRNA pool. According to the experimental estimations of circulating placental miRNAs [172] and mathematical modeling [173], the tumors should reach a considerable size (0.3–0.6 g) before tumor miRNAs could reach the detection threshold in plasma. A lack of cancer-specific miRNAs, small tumor biomass early in disease, and the dilution of tissue-specific miRNAs in circulation may hinder the early detection of tumor-derived circulating miRNAs. Given the promise of miRNAs as noninvasive clinical biomarkers, different strategies have been suggested to overcome these limitations early in disease, when the detection of tumors is most desirable [174]. Circulating miRNAs are primarily associated with Argonaute complexes, and a minor part of circulating miRNA is contained within extracellular vesicles (EVs) [175]. EVs are shed in a highly regulated manner from their cells of origin and are reported to have disease unique signatures of nucleic acids [176]. Therefore, the selective detection of EV-associated circulating miRNAs could prove valuable in enriching the low abundant tissue-specific circulating miRNAs [174].

Despite the exponential increase in the number of studies on circulating miRNAs as disease biomarkers over the last years, circulating miRNAs are in the infancy toward becoming highly specific clinical biomarkers. Many circulating miRNAs, identified as potential disease biomarkers, are associated with a variety of diseases. Furthermore, reported miRNA profiles for a given disease significantly differ between different studies. This can be in part attributed to the current methodological limitations for detecting low level circulating miRNAs, as well as to the preanalytical and the heterogeneity of studied cohorts.

Preanalytical variables during collection and processing of blood to obtain cell-free, circulating miRNAs may significantly affect the levels of circulating miRNAs as excellently reviewed by Nair *et al.* [177]. Therefore, all the study samples should be obtained in the same way, using standard operating procedure for sample collection and processing to minimize the preanalytical variability in circulating miRNA detection. An important source of the preanalytical variability, that considerably affect circulating miRNA levels, is the contamination of circulating cell-free miRNAs with cellular miRNAs, originating from epithelial cells at the site of skin puncture, red blood cell hemolysis releasing a large amount of contaminating miRNAs, as well as from contaminating monocytes and/or platelets. Such cellular contamination could be minimized by discarding first milliliters of withdrawn blood, using a larger-gauge needle, minimizing tourniquet use, using adequate centrifugation speed and preparing platelet-free plasma (reviewed in [177]). Several miRNAs have been identified, which can estimate the contribution of different cellular contaminants, such as platelets or red blood cell lysis, to the plasma miRNA profile [178, 179]. In addition, study subjects have to be matched for age, sex, smoking history, and end-stage organ dysfunction, or miRNA levels have to be adjusted for these confounders, known to significantly affect miRNA levels (reviewed in [177]).

To measure circulating miRNA levels, several methods could be used, including quantitative PCR, high-density microarray technology or next generation sequencing. When using plasma as a source biofluid for circulating miRNA detection heparin should be avoided as it may inhibit qPCR. Another critical step in the analysis of circulating miRNA is data normalization, which is rather challenging when compared to the analysis of cellular and tissue miRNA expression. Normalization strategies significantly vary across the published studies on circulating miRNAs, further contributing to analytical variability. In contrast to the measurement of cellular miRNAs, there is no optimal housekeeping gene for normalization of circulating RNA levels, and a global median normalization can be used as a normalization method.

http://dx.doi.org/10.5772/61551

The simplest method to normalize circulating miRNA levels is to use the defined plasma volume, from which RNA is isolated, combined with the "Spike In" exogenous miRNA controls. The use of "Spike In" exogenous miRNA controls, derived, e.g., from *Caenorhabditis elegans* (cel-miR-39), is highly recommended during the isolation of RNA from plasma or serum as quality control for the technical variation arising from variations in RNA isolation, and the differential efficiencies of the reverse transcription and real-time PCR [179, 180].

Up to date, no reports exist on investigating the circulating levels of miRNAs in APS patients. Nevertheless, the down-regulation of tissue factor-targeting miRNAs, miR-19b, and miR-20a in peripheral blood monocytes from SLE and APS patients as compared to healthy controls inversely correlated with the surface tissue factor expression on monocytes and may contribute to the increased thrombosis risk in APS and SLE patients [181]. Circulating miRNAs may prove valuable as biomarkers in APS, in particular in patients with obstetric APS and APS-related placental dysfunction. Human placenta is a relatively large, well-perfused organ, present only during pregnancy, which makes it an excellent solid tissue model, very likely to contribute to the pool of circulating miRNAs. During pregnancy, placenta-specific miRNAs are detected in maternal circulation. Many of these miRNAs exhibit strict placental specificity and cannot be detected in paternal circulation or plasma of nonpregnant control women [172]. Specifically, the characterization of circulating and placental miRNAs by small RNA deep sequencing showed strong 5240-fold and 28-fold enrichment of the miR-498 cluster in placentas and maternal plasma, respectively, as compared to paternal plasma. This indicated strong, tissue-specific contribution of placenta to the maternal circulating miRNA pool. Furthermore, placental miRNA fingerprints, including miR-498 cluster isomiRs, were sufficiently unique between the subjects to enable matching of the maternal plasma sample to its specific source placenta. This suggests that clinically relevant alterations of placental miRNAs may be present in maternal plasma of women with pregnancy complications, such as preeclampsia or obstetric APS. Such miRNAs could serve as noninvasive biomarkers of placental disease in obstetric APS, allowing for its better monitoring and on time intervention.

5. Conclusion

The classification of APS is based on three aPL laboratory tests that need to be positive in addition to its clinical manifestations. Both the clinical spectrum of APS and the serological markers are more polymorphic than it was thought in the past. Additional laboratory tests have been proposed in order to improve the diagnostic and predictive power, but promising results have been reported especially for anti-β_2GPI-DI and anti-PS/PT antibodies. Discovering new markers did not ease the recognition of patients with APS, and therefore modern trends propose the determination of multiple classes of aPL to gain a common score, which could estimate the risk for arterial/venous thrombosis in APS patients. Risk stratification itself represents a major challenge. However, the potential roles of aPL (as a risk or even as a prognostic factor for arterial/venous thrombosis and miscarriages) will occupy future debates.

Author details

Polona Žigon[1], Mojca Božič-Mijovski[2], Mojca Frank Bertoncelj[3], Aleš Ambrožič[1], Matija Tomšič[1], Alojzija Hočevar[1], Borut Božič[1,4], Snežna Sodin Šemrl[1,5], Tanja Kveder[1] and Saša Čučnik[1,4*]

*Address all correspondence to: sasa.cucnik@guest.arnes.si

1 Department of Rheumatology, University Medical Centre Ljubljana, Ljubljana, Slovenia

2 Department of Vascular Diseases, University Medical Centre Ljubljana, Ljubljana, Slovenia

3 Center of Experimental Rheumatology, University Hospital Zurich, Zurich, Switzerland

4 Faculty of Pharmacy, Chair for Clinical Biochemistry, University of Ljubljana, Ljubljana, Slovenia

5 Faculty of Mathematics, Natural Science and Information Technology, University of Primorska, Koper, Slovenia

References

[1] Hughes GR. Thrombosis, abortion, cerebral disease, and the lupus anticoagulant. British Medical Journal (Clinical Research Ed). 1983;287(6399):1088–9.

[2] Cervera R, Piette JC, Font J, Khamashta MA, Shoenfeld Y, Camps MT, et al. Antiphospholipid syndrome: clinical and immunologic manifestations and patterns of disease expression in a cohort of 1,000 patients. Arthritis and Rheumatism. 2002;46(4):1019–27.

[3] de Groot PG, Lutters B, Derksen RH, Lisman T, Meijers JC, Rosendaal FR. Lupus anticoagulants and the risk of a first episode of deep venous thrombosis. Journal of Thrombosis and Haemostasis. 2005;3(9):1993–7.

[4] Galli M, Luciani D, Bertolini G, Barbui T. Lupus anticoagulants are stronger risk factors for thrombosis than anticardiolipin antibodies in the antiphospholipid syndrome: a systematic review of the literature. Blood. 2003;101(5):1827–32.

[5] Cervera R, Khamashta MA, Shoenfeld Y, Camps MT, Jacobsen S, Kiss E, et al. Morbidity and mortality in the antiphospholipid syndrome during a 5-year period: a multicentre prospective study of 1000 patients. Annals of the Rheumatic Diseases. 2009;68(9): 1428–32.

[6] Asherson RA, Cervera R, de Groot PG, Erkan D, Boffa MC, Piette JC, et al. Catastrophic antiphospholipid syndrome: international consensus statement on classification criteria and treatment guidelines. Lupus. 2003;12(7):530–4.

[7] Asherson RA, Cervera R, Piette JC, Font J, Lie JT, Burcoglu A, et al. Catastrophic antiphospholipid syndrome. Clinical and laboratory features of 50 patients. Medicine. 1998;77(3):195–207.

[8] Asherson RA, Espinosa G, Cervera R, Font J, Reverter JC. Catastrophic antiphospholipid syndrome: proposed guidelines for diagnosis and treatment. Journal of Clinical Rheumatology: Practical Reports on Rheumatic & Musculoskeletal Diseases. 2002;8(3):157–65.

[9] Cervera R, Bucciarelli S, Plasin MA, Gomez-Puerta JA, Plaza J, Pons-Estel G, et al. Catastrophic antiphospholipid syndrome (CAPS): descriptive analysis of a series of 280 patients from the "CAPS Registry." Journal of Autoimmunity. 2009;32(3–4):240–5.

[10] Bucciarelli S, Espinosa G, Cervera R, Erkan D, Gomez-Puerta JA, Ramos-Casals M, et al. Mortality in the catastrophic antiphospholipid syndrome: causes of death and prognostic factors in a series of 250 patients. Arthritis and Rheumatism. 2006;54(8): 2568–76.

[11] Miyakis S, Lockshin MD, Atsumi T, Branch DW, Brey RL, Cervera R, et al. International consensus statement on an update of the classification criteria for definite antiphospholipid syndrome (APS). Journal of Thrombosis and Haemostasis. 2006;4(2): 295–306.

[12] Wilson WA, Gharavi AE, Koike T, Lockshin MD, Branch DW, Piette JC, et al. International consensus statement on preliminary classification criteria for definite antiphospholipid syndrome: report of an international workshop. Arthritis and Rheumatism. 1999;42(7):1309–11.

[13] Pierangeli SS, de Groot PG, Dlott J, Favaloro E, Harris EN, Lakos G, et al. 'Criteria' aPL tests: report of a task force and preconference workshop at the 13th International Congress on Antiphospholipid Antibodies, Galveston, Texas, April 2010. Lupus. 2011;20(2):182–90.

[14] Sciascia S, Sanna G, Murru V, Roccatello D, Khamashta MA, Bertolaccini ML. Antiprothrombin (aPT) and anti-phosphatidylserine/prothrombin (aPS/PT) antibodies and the risk of thrombosis in the antiphospholipid syndrome. A systematic review. Thrombosis and Haemostasis. 2013;111(2).

[15] Zigon P, Cucnik S, Ambrozic A, Kveder T, Semrl SS, Rozman B, et al. Detection of antiphosphatidylserine/prothrombin antibodies and their potential diagnostic value. Clinical and Developmental Immunology. 2013;2013:8.

[16] Otomo K, Atsumi T, Amengual O, Fujieda Y, Kato M, Oku K, et al. Efficacy of the antiphospholipid score for the diagnosis of antiphospholipid syndrome and its predictive value for thrombotic events. Arthritis and Rheumatism. 2012;64(2):504–12.

[17] Sciascia S, Sanna G, Murru V, Roccatello D, Khamashta MA, Bertolaccini ML. GAPSS: the Global Anti-phospholipid Syndrome Score. Rheumatology (Oxford). 2013;52(8):1397–403.

[18] Bozic B, Cucnik S, Gaspersic N, Ambrozic A, Kveder T, Rozman B. Rational laboratory diagnostics of antiphospholipid antibodies: anti-cardiolipin, anti-á2-glycoprotein I, anti-prothrombin and anti-annexin v antibodies. Journal of the International Federation of Clinical Chemistry. 2010;20(4).

[19] Andreoli L, Tincani A. Beyond the "syndrome": antiphospholipid antibodies as risk factors. Arthritis and Rheumatism. 2012;64(2):342–5.

[20] Hernandez-Molina G, Espericueta-Arriola G, Cabral AR. The role of lupus anticoagulant and triple marker positivity as risk factors for rethrombosis in patients with primary antiphospholipid syndrome. Clinical and Experimental Rheumatology. 2013;31(3):382–8.

[21] Pengo V, Ruffatti A, Legnani C, Gresele P, Barcellona D, Erba N, et al. Clinical course of high-risk patients diagnosed with antiphospholipid syndrome. Journal of Thrombosis and Haemostasis. 2010;8(2):237–42.

[22] Roggenbuck D, Egerer K, von Landenberg P, Hiemann R, Feist E, Burmester GR, et al. Antiphospholipid antibody profiling: time for a new technical approach? Autoimmunity Reviews. 2012;11(11):821–6.

[23] Pierangeli SS, Silva LK, Harris EN. A flow cytometric assay for the detection of antiphospholipid antibodies. American Clinical Laboratory. 1999;18(6):18–9.

[24] Tozzoli R, Villalta D. Autoantibody profiling of patients with antiphospholipid syndrome using an automated multiplexed immunoassay system. Autoimmunity Reviews. 2014;13(1):59–63.

[25] Qin J, Liang H, Shi D, Dai J, Xu Z, Chen D, et al. A panel of microRNAs as a new biomarkers for the detection of deep vein thrombosis. Journal of Thrombosis and Thrombolysis. 2014; 39(2): 215-21.

[26] Hu Y, Liu CM, Qi L, He TZ, Shi-Guo L, Hao CJ, et al. Two common SNPs in pri-miR-125a alter the mature miRNA expression and associate with recurrent pregnancy loss in a Han-Chinese population. RNA Biology. 2011;8(5):861–72.

[27] Jeon YJ, Choi YS, Rah H, Kim SY, Choi DH, Cha SH, et al. Association study of microRNA polymorphisms with risk of idiopathic recurrent spontaneous abortion in Korean women. Gene. 2012;494(2):168–73.

[28] Bertolaccini ML, Amengual O, Andreoli L, Atsumi T, Chighizola CB, Forastiero R, et al. 14th International Congress on Antiphospholipid Antibodies Task Force. Report on antiphospholipid syndrome laboratory diagnostics and trends. Autoimmunity Reviews. 2014;13(9):917–30.

[29] Bertolaccini ML, Amengual O, Atsumi T, Binder WL, de LB, Forastiero R, et al. 'Non-criteria' aPL tests: report of a task force and preconference workshop at the 13th International Congress on Antiphospholipid Antibodies, Galveston, TX, USA, April 2010. Lupus. 2011;20(2):191–205.

[30] Favaloro EJ, Wong RC. Antiphospholipid antibody testing for the antiphospholipid syndrome: a comprehensive practical review including a synopsis of challenges and recent guidelines. Pathology. 2014;46(6):481–95.

[31] Roubey RA. Risky business: the interpretation, use, and abuse of antiphospholipid antibody tests in clinical practice. Lupus. 2010;19(4):440–5.

[32] Pengo V, Banzato A, Bison E, Bracco A, Denas G, Ruffatti A. What have we learned about antiphospholipid syndrome from patients and antiphospholipid carrier cohorts? Seminars in Thrombosis and Hemostasis. 2012;38(4):322–7.

[33] Galli M. Interpretation and recommended testing for antiphospholipid antibodies. Seminars in Thrombosis and Hemostasis. 2012;38(4):348–52.

[34] Meroni PL, Chighizola CB, Rovelli F, Gerosa M. Antiphospholipid syndrome in 2014: more clinical manifestations, novel pathogenic players and emerging biomarkers. Arthritis Research and Therapy. 2014;16(2):209.

[35] Pengo V, Ruffatti A, Legnani C, Testa S, Fierro T, Marongiu F, et al. Incidence of a first thromboembolic event in asymptomatic carriers of high-risk antiphospholipid antibody profile: a multicenter prospective study. Blood. 2011;118(17):4714–8.

[36] Ruffatti A, Tonello M, Visentin MS, Bontadi A, Hoxha A, De Carolis S, et al. Risk factors for pregnancy failure in patients with anti-phospholipid syndrome treated with conventional therapies: a multicentre, case–control study. Rheumatology (Oxford). 2011;50(9):1684–9.

[37] de Groot PG, Derksen RH. Pathophysiology of the antiphospholipid syndrome. Journal of Thrombosis and Haemostasis. 2005;3(8):1854–60.

[38] Brandt JT, Triplett DA, Alving B, Scharrer I. Criteria for the diagnosis of lupus anticoagulants: an update. On behalf of the Subcommittee on Lupus Anticoagulant/Antiphospholipid Antibody of the Scientific and Standardisation Committee of the ISTH. Thrombosis and Haemostasis. 1995;74(4):1185–90.

[39] Exner T, Triplett DA, Taberner D, Machin SJ. Guidelines for testing and revised criteria for lupus anticoagulants. SSC Subcommittee for the Standardization of Lupus Anticoagulants. Thrombosis and Haemostasis. 1991;65(3):320–2.

[40] Pengo V, Tripodi A, Reber G, Rand JH, Ortel TL, Galli M, et al. Update of the guidelines for lupus anticoagulant detection. Subcommittee on Lupus Anticoagulant/Antiphospholipid Antibody of the Scientific and Standardisation Committee of the International Society on Thrombosis and Haemostasis. Journal of Thrombosis and Haemostasis. 2009;7(10):1737–40.

[41] Scientific Standardization Subcommittee (2014); Laboratory Testing for the Lupus Anticoagulant. CLSI document H60-A: 116, 4.4.2014

[42] Moore GW. Commonalities and contrasts in recent guidelines for lupus anticoagulant detection. International Journal of Laboratory Hematology. 2014;36(3):364–73.

[43] Favaloro EJ. Preanalytical variables in coagulation testing. Blood Coagulation and Fibrinolysis. 2007;18(1):86–9.

[44] Pengo V, Tripodi A, Reber G, Rand JH, Ortel TL, Galli M, et al. Update of the guidelines for lupus anticoagulant detection. Subcommittee on Lupus Anticoagulant/Antiphospholipid Antibody of the Scientific and Standardisation Committee of the International Society on Thrombosis and Haemostasis. Journal of Thrombosis and Haemostasis. 2009;7(10):1737–40.

[45] Reber G, Meijer P. In ECAT veritas? Lupus. 2012;21(7):722–4.

[46] Devreese KM. No more mixing tests required for integrated assay systems in the laboratory diagnosis of lupus anticoagulants? Journal of Thrombosis and Haemostasis. 2010;8(5):1120–2.

[47] Roubey RA. Immunology of the antiphospholipid antibody syndrome. Arthritis and Rheumatism. 1996;39(9):1444–54.

[48] Rand JH, Wolgast LR. Dos and don'ts in diagnosing antiphospholipid syndrome. Hematology/the Education Program of the American Society of Hematology American Society of Hematology Education Program. 2012;2012:455–9.

[49] Bozic B, Kveder T, Stegnar M, Morosini-Berus E, Kos-Golja M, Peternel P, et al. Influence of degraded phosphatidylserine on binding of antiphospholipid antibodies. International Archives of Allergy and Immunology. 1997;112(1):19–26.

[50] Loizou S, McCrea JD, Rudge JC, Reynolds R, Boyle CC, Harris EN. Measurement of anticardiolipin antibodies by an enzyme-linked immunosorbent assay (ELISA). Standardization and quantitation of results. Clinical and Experimental Rheumatology. 1985(2):738–45.

[51] Willems GM, Janssen MP, Pelsers MM, Comfurius P, Galli M, Zwaal RF, et al. Role of divalency in the high-affinity binding of anticardiolipin antibody-beta 2-glycoprotein I complexes to lipid membranes. Biochemistry. 1996;35(43):13833–42.

[52] Bozic B, Kveder T, Stegnar M, Morosini-Berus E, Kos-Golja M, Peternel P, et al. Influence of degraded phosphatidylserine on binding of antiphospholipid antibodies. International Archives of Allergy and Immunology. 1997;112(1):19–26.

[53] Harris EN. Special report. The Second International Anti-cardiolipin Standardization Workshop/the Kingston Anti-Phospholipid Antibody Study (KAPS) group. American Journal of Clinical Pathology. 1990;94(4):476–84.

[54] Harris EN, Chan JK, Asherson RA, Aber VR, Gharavi AE, Hughes GR. Thrombosis, recurrent fetal loss, and thrombocytopenia. Predictive value of the anticardiolipin antibody test. Archives of Internal Medicine. 1986;146(11):2153–6.

[55] Harris EN, Gharavi AE, Patel SP, Hughes GR. Evaluation of the anti-cardiolipin antibody test: report of an international workshop held 4 April 1986. Clinical and Experimental Immunology. 1987;68(1):215–22.

[56] Harris EN, Pierangeli S, Birch D. Anticardiolipin wet workshop report. Fifth International Symposium on antiphospholipid antibodies. American Journal of Clinical Pathology. 1994;101(5):616–24.

[57] Pierangeli SS, Stewart M, Silva LK, Harris EN. An antiphospholipid wet workshop: 7th International Symposium on Antiphospholipid Antibodies. Journal of Rheumatology. 1998;25(1):156–60.

[58] Lakos G, Favaloro EJ, Harris EN, Meroni PL, Tincani A, Wong RC, et al. International consensus guidelines on anticardiolipin and anti-beta2-glycoprotein I testing: report from the 13th International Congress on Antiphospholipid Antibodies. Arthritis and Rheumatism. 2012;64(1):1–10.

[59] Pierangeli SS, Favaloro EJ, Lakos G, Meroni PL, Tincani A, Wong RC, et al. Standards and reference materials for the anticardiolipin and anti-beta2glycoprotein I assays: a report of recommendations from the APL Task Force at the 13th International Congress on Antiphospholipid Antibodies. Clinica Chimica Acta; International Journal of Clinical Chemistry. 2012;413(1–2):358–60.

[60] Audrain MA, Colonna F, Morio F, Hamidou MA, Muller JY. Comparison of different kits in the detection of autoantibodies to cardiolipin and beta2glycoprotein 1. Rheumatology (Oxford). 2004;43(2):181–5.

[61] Devreese K, Hoylaerts MF. Challenges in the diagnosis of the antiphospholipid syndrome. Clinical Chemistry. 2010;56(6):930–40.

[62] Marai I, Tincani A, Balestrieri G, Shoenfeld Y. Anticardiolipin and anti-beta-2-glycoprotein I antibodies. Autoimmunity. 2005;38(1):33–8.

[63] de Laat B, Mertens K, de Groot PG. Mechanisms of disease: antiphospholipid antibodies-from clinical association to pathologic mechanism. Nature Clinical Practice. Rheumatology. 2008;4(4):192–9.

[64] Lin F, Murphy R, White B, Kelly J, Feighery C, Doyle R, et al. Circulating levels of beta2-glycoprotein I in thrombotic disorders and in inflammation. Lupus. 2006;15(2): 87–93.

[65] Horstman LL, Jy W, Bidot CJ, Ahn YS, Kelley RE, Zivadinov R, et al. Antiphospholipid antibodies: paradigm in transition. Journal of Neuroinflammation. 2009;6:3.

[66] Ragusa MA, Costa S, Cefalu AB, Noto D, Fayer F, Travali S, et al. RT-PCR and in situ hybridization analysis of apolipoprotein H expression in rat normal tissues. International Journal of Molecular Medicine. 2006;18(3):449–55.

[67] Lozier J, Takahashi N, Putnam FW. Complete amino acid sequence of human plasma beta 2-glycoprotein I. Proceedings of the National Academy of Sciences of the United States of America. 1984;81(12):3640–4.

[68] Hunt JE, Simpson RJ, Krilis SA. Identification of a region of beta 2-glycoprotein I critical for lipid binding and anti-cardiolipin antibody cofactor activity. Proceedings of the National Academy of Sciences of the United States of America. 1993;90(6):2141–5.

[69] Schwarzenbacher R, Zeth K, Diederichs K, Gries A, Kostner GM, Laggner P, et al. Crystal structure of human beta2-glycoprotein I: implications for phospholipid binding and the antiphospholipid syndrome. EMBO Journal. 1999;18(22):6228–39.

[70] Sodin-Semrl S, Frank M, Ambrožič A, Pavlič J, Šuštar V, Čučnik S, et al. Interactions of phospholipid binding proteins with negatively charged membranes: β2-glycoprotein I as a model mechanism. In: Leitmannova Liu A, editor. Advances in Planar Lipid Bilayers and Liposomes. 8. 1st ed. Amsterdam: Elsevier; 2008. pp 243–73.

[71] Agar C, van Os GM, Morgelin M, Sprenger RR, Marquart JA, Urbanus RT, et al. Beta2-glycoprotein I can exist in 2 conformations: implications for our understanding of the antiphospholipid syndrome. Blood. 2010;116(8):1336–43.

[72] Bouma B, de Groot PG, van den Elsen JM, Ravelli RB, Schouten A, Simmelink MJ, et al. Adhesion mechanism of human beta(2)-glycoprotein I to phospholipids based on its crystal structure. EMBO Journal. 1999;18(19):5166–74.

[73] Hammel M, Kriechbaum M, Gries A, Kostner GM, Laggner P, Prassl R. Solution structure of human and bovine beta(2)-glycoprotein I revealed by small-angle X-ray scattering. Journal of Molecular Biology. 2002;321(1):85–97.

[74] de Laat B, Derksen RH, van Lummel M, Pennings MT, de Groot PG. Pathogenic anti-beta2-glycoprotein I antibodies recognize domain I of beta2-glycoprotein I only after a conformational change. Blood. 2006;107(5):1916–24.

[75] Wang MX, Kandiah DA, Ichikawa K, Khamashta M, Hughes G, Koike T, et al. Epitope specificity of monoclonal anti-beta 2-glycoprotein I antibodies derived from patients with the antiphospholipid syndrome. Journal of Immunology. 1995;155(3): 1629–36.

[76] Kasahara H, Matsuura E, Kaihara K, Yamamoto D, Kobayashi K, Inagaki J, et al. Antigenic structures recognized by anti-beta2-glycoprotein I auto-antibodies. International Immunology. 2005;17(12):1533–42.

[77] Mahler M, Norman GL, Meroni PL, Khamashta M. Autoantibodies to domain 1 of beta 2 glycoprotein 1: a promising candidate biomarker for risk management in antiphospholipid syndrome. Autoimmunity Reviews. 2012;12(2):313–7.

[78] Ambrozic A, Avicin T, Ichikawa K, Kveder T, Matsuura E, Hojnik M, et al. Anti-beta(2)-glycoprotein I antibodies in children with atopic dermatitis. International Immunology. 2002;14(7):823–30.

[79] Cucnik S, Kveder T, Krizaj I, Rozman B, Bozic B. High avidity anti-beta 2-glycoprotein I antibodies in patients with antiphospholipid syndrome. Annals of the Rheumatic Diseases. 2004;63(11):1478–82.

[80] de Laat B, Derksen RH, de Groot PG. High-avidity anti-beta2 glycoprotein I antibodies highly correlate with thrombosis in contrast to low-avidity anti-beta2 glycoprotein I antibodies. Journal of Thrombosis and Haemostasis. 2006;4(7):1619–21.

[81] Zager U, Irman S, Lunder M, Skarabot M, Musevic I, Hodnik V, et al. Immunochemical properties and pathological relevance of anti-beta2-glycoprotein I antibodies of different avidity. International Immunology. 2011;23(8):511–8.

[82] Zager U, Lunder M, Čučnik S, Kveder T, Rozman B, Božič B. Immunodominant epitopes of beta2-glycoprotein I for high avidity antibodies. 8th International Congress on Autoimmunity; May 9–13; Granada, Spain: Geneva: Kenes International; 2012.

[83] Meroni PL, Borghi MO, Raschi E, Tedesco F. Pathogenesis of antiphospholipid syndrome: understanding the antibodies. Nature Reviews. Rheumatology. 2011;7(6): 330–9.

[84] Blank M, Shoenfeld Y, Cabilly S, Heldman Y, Fridkin M, Katchalski-Katzir E. Prevention of experimental antiphospholipid syndrome and endothelial cell activation by synthetic peptides. Proceedings of the National Academy of Sciences of the United States of America. 1999;96(9):5164–8.

[85] Cucnik S, Kveder T, Artenjak A, Ulcova Gallova Z, Swadzba J, Musial J, et al. Avidity of anti-beta2-glycoprotein I antibodies in patients with antiphospholipid syndrome. Lupus. 2012;21(7):764–5.

[86] Iverson GM, von Muhlen CA, Staub HL, Lassen AJ, Binder W, Norman GL. Patients with atherosclerotic syndrome, negative in anti-cardiolipin assays, make IgA autoantibodies that preferentially target domain 4 of beta2-GPI. Journal of Autoimmunity. 2006;27(4):266–71.

[87] de Laat B, Derksen RH, Urbanus RT, de Groot PG. IgG antibodies that recognize epitope Gly40-Arg43 in domain I of beta 2-glycoprotein I cause LAC, and their presence correlates strongly with thrombosis. Blood. 2005;105(4):1540–5.

[88] Giannakopoulos B, Passam F, Ioannou Y, Krilis SA. How we diagnose the antiphospholipid syndrome. Blood. 2009;113(5):985–94.

[89] Cucnik S, Bozic B, Kveder T, Tomsic M, Rozman B. Avidity of anti-beta2-glycoprotein I and thrombosis or pregnancy loss in patients with antiphospholipid syndrome. Annals of the New York Academy of Sciences. 2005;1051:141–7.

[90] Cucnik S, Kveder T, Ulcova-Gallova Z, Swadzba J, Musial J, Valesini G, et al. The avidity of anti-beta2-glycoprotein I antibodies in patients with or without antiphospholipid syndrome: a collaborative study in the frame of the European forum on antiphospholipid antibodies. Lupus. 2011;20(11):1166–71.

[91] Artenjak A, Kozelj M, Lakota K, Cucnik S, Bozic B, Sodin-Semrl S. High avidity anti-b2-glycoprotein I antibodies activate human coronary artery endothelial cells and trigger peripheral blood mononuclear cell migration. European Journal of Inflammation. 2013;11(2):385–96.

[92] Zager U, Kveder T, Cucnik S, Bozic B, Lunder M. Anti-beta2-glycoprotein I paratopes and beta2-glycoprotein I epitopes characterization using random peptide libraries. Autoimmunity. 2014;47(7):438–44.

[93] Wong RC, Favaloro EJ, Adelstein S, Baumgart K, Bird R, Brighton TA, et al. Consensus guidelines on anti-beta 2 glycoprotein I testing and reporting. Pathology. 2008;40(1):58–63.

[94] Artenjak A, Leonardi A, Krizaj I, Ambrozic A, Sodin-Semrl S, Bozic B, et al. Optimization of unnicked beta2-glycoprotein I and high avidity anti-beta2-glycoprotein I antibodies isolation. Journal of Immunology Research. 2014;2014:195687.

[95] Pengo V, Biasiolo A, Fior MG. Autoimmune antiphospholipid antibodies are directed against a cryptic epitope expressed when beta 2-glycoprotein I is bound to a suitable surface. Thrombosis and Haemostasis. 1995;73(1):29–34.

[96] Meroni PL, Biggioggero M, Pierangeli SS, Sheldon J, Zegers I, Borghi MO. Standardization of autoantibody testing: a paradigm for serology in rheumatic diseases. Nature Reviews. Rheumatology. 2014;10(1):35–43.

[97] Willis R, Grossi C, Orietta Borghi M, Martos-Sevilla G, Zegers I, Sheldon J, et al. International standards for IgG and IgM anti-beta2glycoprotein antibody measurement. Lupus. 2014;23(12):1317–9.

[98] Andreoli L, Fredi M, Nalli C, Piantoni S, Reggia R, Dall'Ara F, et al. Clinical significance of IgA anti-cardiolipin and IgA anti-beta2glycoprotein I antibodies. Current Rheumatology Reports. 2013;15(7):343.

[99] Lakos G, Kiss E, Regeczy N, Tarjan P, Soltesz P, Zeher M, et al. Isotype distribution and clinical relevance of anti-beta2-glycoprotein I (beta2-GPI) antibodies: importance of IgA isotype. Clinical and Experimental Immunology. 1999;117(3):574–9.

[100] Samarkos M, Davies KA, Gordon C, Loizou S. Clinical significance of IgA anticardiolipin and anti-beta2-GP1 antibodies in patients with systemic lupus erythematosus and primary antiphospholipid syndrome. Clinical Rheumatology. 2006;25(2):199–204.

[101] Cucurull E, Gharavi AE, Diri E, Mendez E, Kapoor D, Espinoza LR. IgA anticardiolipin and anti-beta2-glycoprotein I are the most prevalent isotypes in African Ameri-

http://dx.doi.org/10.5772/61551

can patients with systemic lupus erythematosus. American Journal of the Medical Sciences. 1999;318(1):55–60.

[102] Tajima C, Suzuki Y, Mizushima Y, Ichikawa Y. Clinical significance of immunoglobulin A antiphospholipid antibodies: possible association with skin manifestations and small vessel vasculitis. Journal of Rheumatology. 1998;25(9):1730–6.

[103] Molina JF, Gutierrez-Urena S, Molina J, Uribe O, Richards S, De Ceulaer C, et al. Variability of anticardiolipin antibody isotype distribution in 3 geographic populations of patients with systemic lupus erythematosus. Journal of Rheumatology. 1997;24(2): 291–6.

[104] Akhter E, Shums Z, Norman GL, Binder W, Fang H, Petri M. Utility of antiphosphatidylserine/prothrombin and IgA antiphospholipid assays in systemic lupus erythematosus. Journal of Rheumatology. 2013;40(3):282–6.

[105] Despierres L, Beziane A, Kaplanski G, Granel B, Serratrice J, Cohen W, et al. Contribution of anti-beta2glycoprotein I IgA antibodies to the diagnosis of anti-phospholipid syndrome: potential interest of target domains to discriminate thrombotic and non-thrombotic patients. Rheumatology (Oxford). 2014;53(7):1215–8.

[106] Mehrani T, Petri M. Association of IgA Anti-beta2 glycoprotein I with clinical and laboratory manifestations of systemic lupus erythematosus. Journal of Rheumatology. 2011;38(1):64–8.

[107] Petri M, Orbai AM, Alarcon GS, Gordon C, Merrill JT, Fortin PR, et al. Derivation and validation of the Systemic Lupus International Collaborating Clinics classification criteria for systemic lupus erythematosus. Arthritis and Rheumatism. 2012;64(8): 2677–86.

[108] Ruiz-Garcia R, Serrano M, Martinez-Flores JA, Mora S, Morillas L, Martin-Mola MA, et al. Isolated IgA anti- beta2 glycoprotein I antibodies in patients with clinical criteria for antiphospholipid syndrome. Journal of Immunology Research. 2014;2014:704395.

[109] Murthy V, Willis R, Romay-Penabad Z, Ruiz-Limon P, Martinez-Martinez LA, Jatwani S, et al. Value of isolated IgA anti-beta2 -glycoprotein I positivity in the diagnosis of the antiphospholipid syndrome. Arthritis and Rheumatism. 2013;65(12):3186–93.

[110] de Laat B, de Groot PG. Autoantibodies directed against domain I of beta2-glycoprotein I. Current Rheumatology Reports. 2011;13(1):70–6.

[111] Iverson GM, Victoria EJ, Marquis DM. Anti-beta2 glycoprotein I (beta2GPI) autoantibodies recognize an epitope on the first domain of beta2GPI. Proceedings of the National Academy of Sciences of the United States of America. 1998;95(26):15542–6.

[112] Erkan D, Espinosa G, Cervera R. Catastrophic antiphospholipid syndrome: updated diagnostic algorithms. Autoimmunity Reviews. 2010;10(2):74–9.

[113] de Laat B, Pengo V, Pabinger I, Musial J, Voskuyl AE, Bultink IE, et al. The association between circulating antibodies against domain I of beta2-glycoprotein I and thrombosis: an international multicenter study. Journal of Thrombosis and Haemostasis. 2009;7(11):1767–73.

[114] Cousins L, Pericleous C, Khamashta M, Bertolaccini ML, Ioannou Y, Giles I, et al. Antibodies to domain I of beta-2-glycoprotein I and IgA antiphospholipid antibodies in patients with 'seronegative' antiphospholipid syndrome. Annals of Rheumatic Diseases. 2015;74(1):317–9.

[115] Ioannou Y, Romay-Penabad Z, Pericleous C, Giles I, Papalardo E, Vargas G, et al. In vivo inhibition of antiphospholipid antibody-induced pathogenicity utilizing the antigenic target peptide domain I of beta2-glycoprotein I: proof of concept. Journal of Thrombosis and Haemostasis. 2009;7(5):833–42.

[116] Ciesla M, Wypasek E, Undas A. IgA antiphospholipid antibodies and anti-domain 1 of beta 2 glycoprotein 1 antibodies are associated with livedo reticularis and heart valve disease in antiphospholipid syndrome. Advances in Clinical and Experimental Medicine. 2014;23(5):729–33.

[117] Iverson GM, Matsuura E, Victoria EJ, Cockerill KA, Linnik MD. The orientation of beta2GPI on the plate is important for the binding of anti-beta2GPI autoantibodies by ELISA. Journal of Autoimmunity. 2002;18(4):289–97.

[118] Pozzi N, Banzato A, Bettin S, Bison E, Pengo V, De Filippis V. Chemical synthesis and characterization of wild-type and biotinylated N-terminal domain 1–64 of beta2-glycoprotein I. Protein Science. 2010;19(5):1065–78.

[119] Banzato A, Pozzi N, Frasson R, De Filippis V, Ruffatti A, Bison E, et al. Antibodies to domain I of beta(2)glycoprotein I are in close relation to patients risk categories in antiphospholipid syndrome (APS). Thrombosis Research. 2011;128(6):583–6.

[120] Iverson GM, Reddel S, Victoria EJ, Cockerill KA, Wang YX, Marti-Renom MA, et al. Use of single point mutations in domain I of beta 2-glycoprotein I to determine fine antigenic specificity of antiphospholipid autoantibodies. Journal of Immunology. 2002;169(12):7097–103.

[121] Mahler M, Radice A, Yang W, Bentow C, Seaman A, Bianchi L, et al. Development and performance evaluation of novel chemiluminescence assays for detection of anti-PR3 and anti-MPO antibodies. Clinica Chimica Acta. 2012;413(7–8):719–26.

[122] Loeliger A. Prothrombin as a co-factor of the circulating anticoagulant in systemic lupus erythematosus? Thrombosis et Diathesis Haemorrhagica. 1959;3:237–56.

[123] Bajaj SP, Rapaport SI, Barclay S, Herbst KD. Acquired hypoprothrombinemia due to non-neutralizing antibodies to prothrombin: mechanism and management. Blood. 1985;65(6):1538–43.

[124] Edson JR, Vogt JM, Hasegawa DK. Abnormal prothrombin crossed-immunoelectrophoresis in patients with lupus inhibitors. Blood. 1984;64(4):807–16.

[125] Fleck RA, Rapaport SI, Rao LV. Anti-prothrombin antibodies and the lupus anticoagulant. Blood. 1988;72(2):512–9.

[126] Bevers EM, Galli M, Barbui T, Comfurius P, Zwaal RF. Lupus anticoagulant IgG's (LA) are not directed to phospholipids only, but to a complex of lipid-bound human prothrombin. Thrombosis and Haemostasis. 1991;66(6):629–32.

[127] Oosting JD, Derksen RH, Bobbink IW, Hackeng TM, Bouma BN, De Groot PG. Antiphospholipid antibodies directed against a combination of phospholipids with prothrombin, protein C, or protein S: an explanation for their pathogenic mechanism? Blood. 1993;81(10):2618–25.

[128] Amengual O, Atsumi T, Koike T. Specificities, properties, and clinical significance of antiprothrombin antibodies. Arthritis and Rheumatism. 2003;48(4):886–95.

[129] Bajaj SP, Rapaport SI, Fierer DS, Herbst KD, Schwartz DB. A mechanism for the hypoprothrombinemia of the acquired hypoprothrombinemia-lupus anticoagulant syndrome. Blood. 1983;61(4):684–92.

[130] Galli M, Bevers EM, Comfurius P, Barbui T, Zwaal RF. Effect of antiphospholipid antibodies on procoagulant activity of activated platelets and platelet-derived microvesicles. British Journal of Haematology. 1993;83(3):466–72.

[131] Arvieux J, Darnige L, Caron C, Reber G, Bensa JC, Colomb MG. Development of an ELISA for autoantibodies to prothrombin showing their prevalence in patients with lupus anticoagulants. Thrombosis and Haemostasis. 1995;74(4):1120–5.

[132] Galli M, Barbui T. Antiprothrombin antibodies: detection and clinical significance in the antiphospholipid syndrome. Blood. 1999;93(7):2149–57.

[133] Matsuura E, Igarashi Y, Yasuda T, Triplett DA, Koike T. Anticardiolipin antibodies recognize beta 2-glycoprotein I structure altered by interacting with an oxygen modified solid phase surface. Journal of Experimental Medicine. 1994;179(2):457–62.

[134] Pengo V, Biasiolo A, Fior MG. Autoimmune antiphospholipid antibodies are directed against a cryptic epitope expressed when beta 2-glycoprotein I is bound to a suitable surface. Thrombosis and Haemostasis. 1995;73(1):29-34.

[135] Cucnik S, Kveder T, Rozman B, Bozic B. Binding of high-avidity anti-beta2-glycoprotein I antibodies. Rheumatology (Oxford). 2004;43(11):1353–6.

[136] Matsuda J, Saitoh N, Gotoh M, Kawasugi K, Gohchi K, Tsukamoto M. Phosphatidyl serine-dependent antiprothrombin antibody is exclusive to patients with lupus anticoagulant. British Journal of Rheumatology. 1996;35(6):589–91.

[137] Galli M, Beretta G, Daldossi M, Bevers EM, Barbui T. Different anticoagulant and immunological properties of anti-prothrombin antibodies in patients with antiphospholipid antibodies. Thrombosis and Haemostasis. 1997;77(3):486–91.

[138] Atsumi T, Ieko M, Bertolaccini ML, Ichikawa K, Tsutsumi A, Matsuura E, et al. Association of autoantibodies against the phosphatidylserine-prothrombin complex with manifestations of the antiphospholipid syndrome and with the presence of lupus anticoagulant. Arthritis and Rheumatism. 2000;43(9):1982–93.

[139] Zigon P, Ambrozic A, Cucnik S, Kveder T, Rozman B, Bozic B. Modified phosphatidylserine-dependent antiprothrombin ELISA enables identification of patients negative for other antiphospholipid antibodies and also detects low avidity antibodies. Clinical Chemistry and Laboratory Medicine. 2011;49(9):1573.

[140] Zigon P, Cucnik S, Ambrozic A, Sodin Semrl S, Kveder T, Bozic B. Antibodies to phosphatidylserine/prothrombin complex as an additional diagnostic marker of APS? Lupus. 2012;21(7):790–2.

[141] Tincani A, Morozzi G, Afeltra A, Alessandri C, Allegri F, Bistoni O, et al. Antiprothrombin antibodies: a comparative analysis of homemade and commercial methods. A collaborative study by the Forum Interdisciplinare per la Ricerca nelle Malattie Autoimmuni (FIRMA). Clinical and Experimental Rheumatology. 2007;25(2):268–74.

[142] Sciascia S, Sanna G, Murru V, Khamashta MA, Bertolaccini ML. Validation of a commercially available kit to detect anti-phosphatidylserine/prothrombin antibodies in a cohort of systemic lupus erythematosus patients. Thrombosis Research. 2014;133(3): 451–4.

[143] Galli M. Anti-Prothrombin Antibodies. In: Asherson RA, Cervera R, Piette JC, Shoenfeld Y, editors. The Antiphospholipid Syndrome II: Elsevier; 2002. p. 59–70.

[144] Bardin N, Alessi MC, Dignat-George F, Vague IJ, Sampol J, Harle JR, et al. Does the anti-prothrombin antibodies measurement provide additional information in patients with thrombosis? Immunobiology. 2007;212(7):557–65.

[145] Nojima J, Iwatani Y, Suehisa E, Kuratsune H, Kanakura Y. The presence of anti-phosphatidylserine/prothrombin antibodies as risk factor for both arterial and venous thrombosis in patients with systemic lupus erythematosus. Haematologica. 2006;91(5):699–702.

[146] Tsutsumi A, Hayashi T, Chino Y, Mamura M, Goto D, Matsumoto I, et al. Significance of antiprothrombin antibodies in patients with systemic lupus erythematosus: clinical evaluation of the antiprothrombin assay and the antiphosphatidylserine/prothrombin assay, and comparison with other antiphospholipid antibody assays. Modern Rheumatology. 2006;16(3):158–64.

[147] Forastiero RR, Martinuzzo ME, Cerrato GS, Kordich LC, Carreras LO. Relationship of anti beta2-glycoprotein I and anti prothrombin antibodies to thrombosis and preg-

nancy loss in patients with antiphospholipid antibodies. Thrombosis and Haemostasis. 1997;78(3):1008–14.

[148] Sater MS, Finan RR, Abu-Hijleh FM, Abu-Hijleh TM, Almawi WY. Anti-phosphatidylserine, anti-cardiolipin, anti-beta2 glycoprotein I and anti-prothrombin antibodies in recurrent miscarriage at 8–12 gestational weeks. European Journal of Obstetrics, Gynecology, and Reproductive Biology. 2012;163(2):170–4.

[149] Sugiura-Ogasawara M, Atsumi T, Ozaki Y, Koike T, Suzumori K. Phosphatidylserine-dependent antiprothrombin antibodies are not useful markers for high-risk women with recurrent miscarriages. Fertility and Sterility. 2004;82(5):1440–2.

[150] Tsutsumi A, Atsumi T, Yamada H, Hirayama KE, Ichikawa K, Fujimoto S, et al. Antiphosphatidylserine/prothrombin antibodies are not frequently found in patients with unexplained recurrent miscarriages. American Journal of Reproductive Immunology. 2001;46(3):242–4.

[151] Akimoto T, Akama T, Saitoh M, Kono I, Sumida T. Antiprothrombin autoantibodies in severe preeclampsia and abortion. American Journal of Medicine. 2001;110(3):188–91.

[152] Bertolaccini ML, Atsumi T, Koike T, Hughes GR, Khamashta MA. Antiprothrombin antibodies detected in two different assay systems. Prevalence and clinical significance in systemic lupus erythematosus. Thrombosis and Haemostasis. 2005;93(2): 289–97.

[153] Marozio L, Curti A, Botta G, Canuto EM, Salton L, Tavella AM, et al. Anti-prothrombin antibodies are associated with adverse pregnancy outcome. American Journal of Reproductive Immunology. 2011;66(5):404–9.

[154] Vlagea A, Gil A, Cuesta MV, Arribas F, Diez J, Lavilla P, et al. Antiphosphatidylserine/prothrombin antibodies (aPS/PT) as potential markers of antiphospholipid syndrome. Clinical and Applied Thrombosis/Hemostasis. 2013;19(3):289–96.

[155] Zigon P, Perdan Pirkmajer K, Tomsic M, Kveder T, Bozic B, Sodin Semrl S, et al. Anti-Phosphatidylserine/Prothrombin Antibodies Are Associated with Adverse Pregnancy Outcomes. Journal of Immunology Research. 2015; 2015: 975704.

[156] Roggenbuck D, Egerer K, Feist E, Burmester GR, Dorner T. Antiphospholipid antibody profiling: association with the clinical phenotype of antiphospholipid syndrome? Comment on the article by Otomo et al. Arthritis and Rheumatism. 2012;64(8):2807–8; author reply 8–9.

[157] Tozzoli R, Villalta D, Kodermaz G, Bagnasco M, Tonutti E, Bizzaro N. Autoantibody profiling of patients with autoimmune thyroid disease using a new multiplexed immunoassay method. Clinical Chemistry and Laboratory Medicine. 2006;44(7):837–42.

[158] Egerer K, Roggenbuck D, Buttner T, Lehmann B, Kohn A, von Landenberg P, et al. Single-step autoantibody profiling in antiphospholipid syndrome using a multi-line dot assay. Arthritis Research and Therapy. 2011;13(4):R118.

[159] Roggenbuck D, Somma V, Schierack P, Borghi MO, Meroni PL. Autoantibody profiling in APS. Lupus. 2014;23(12):1262–4.

[160] Kozomara A, Griffiths-Jones S. miRBase: annotating high confidence microRNAs using deep sequencing data. Nucleic Acids Research. 2014;42(database issue):D68–73.

[161] Chen X, Ba Y, Ma L, Cai X, Yin Y, Wang K, et al. Characterization of microRNAs in serum: a novel class of biomarkers for diagnosis of cancer and other diseases. Cell Research. 2008;18(10):997–1006.

[162] Mitchell PS, Parkin RK, Kroh EM, Fritz BR, Wyman SK, Pogosova-Agadjanyan EL, et al. Circulating microRNAs as stable blood-based markers for cancer detection. Proceedings of the National Academy of Sciences of the United States of America. 2008;105(30):10513–8.

[163] Wang C, Hu J, Lu M, Gu H, Zhou X, Chen X, et al. A panel of five serum miRNAs as a potential diagnostic tool for early-stage renal cell carcinoma. Scientific Reports. 2015;5:7610.

[164] Hansen TF, Carlsen AL, Heegaard NH, Sorensen FB, Jakobsen A. Changes in circulating microRNA-126 during treatment with chemotherapy and bevacizumab predicts treatment response in patients with metastatic colorectal cancer. British Journal of Cancer. 2015;112(4):624–9.

[165] Makino K, Jinnin M, Kajihara I, Honda N, Sakai K, Masuguchi S, et al. Circulating miR-142-3p levels in patients with systemic sclerosis. Clinical and experimental dermatology. 2012;37(1):34–9.

[166] Filkova M, Aradi B, Senolt L, Ospelt C, Vettori S, Mann H, et al. Association of circulating miR-223 and miR-16 with disease activity in patients with early rheumatoid arthritis. Annals of the Rheumatic Diseases. 2014;73(10):1898–904.

[167] Gidlof O, Smith JG, Miyazu K, Gilje P, Spencer A, Blomquist S, et al. Circulating cardio-enriched microRNAs are associated with long-term prognosis following myocardial infarction. BMC Cardiovascular Disorders. 2013;13:12.

[168] Akat KM, Moore-McGriff D, Morozov P, Brown M, Gogakos T, Correa Da Rosa J, et al. Comparative RNA-sequencing analysis of myocardial and circulating small RNAs in human heart failure and their utility as biomarkers. Proceedings of the National Academy of Sciences of the United States of America. 2014;111(30):11151–6.

[169] Qin J, Liang H, Shi D, Dai J, Xu Z, Chen D, et al. A panel of microRNAs as a new biomarkers for the detection of deep vein thrombosis. Journal of Thrombosis and Thrombolysis. 2015;39(2):215–21.

[170] Tsochandaridis M, Nasca L, Toga C, Levy-Mozziconacci A. Circulating MicroRNAs as Clinical Biomarkers in the Predictions of Pregnancy Complications. BioMed Research International. 2015;2015:294954.

[171] Luque A, Farwati A, Crovetto F, Crispi F, Figueras F, Gratacos E, et al. Usefulness of circulating microRNAs for the prediction of early preeclampsia at first-trimester of pregnancy. Scientific Reports. 2014;4:4882.

[172] Williams Z, Ben-Dov IZ, Elias R, Mihailovic A, Brown M, Rosenwaks Z, et al. Comprehensive profiling of circulating microRNA via small RNA sequencing of cDNA libraries reveals biomarker potential and limitations. Proceedings of the National Academy of Sciences of the United States of America. 2013;110(11):4255–60.

[173] Hori SS, Gambhir SS. Mathematical model identifies blood biomarker-based early cancer detection strategies and limitations. Science Translational Medicine. 2011;3(109):109ra16.

[174] Witwer KW. Circulating microRNA biomarker studies: pitfalls and potential solutions. Clinical Chemistry. 2015;61(1):56–63.

[175] Arroyo JD, Chevillet JR, Kroh EM, Ruf IK, Pritchard CC, Gibson DF, et al. Argonaute2 complexes carry a population of circulating microRNAs independent of vesicles in human plasma. Proceedings of the National Academy of Sciences of the United States of America. 2011;108(12):5003–8.

[176] Huang X, Yuan T, Tschannen M, Sun Z, Jacob H, Du M, et al. Characterization of human plasma-derived exosomal RNAs by deep sequencing. BMC Genomics. 2013;14:319.

[177] Nair VS, Pritchard CC, Tewari M, Ioannidis JP. Design and analysis for studying microRNAs in human disease: a primer on -omic technologies. American Journal of Epidemiology. 2014;180(2):140–52.

[178] Kirschner MB, Edelman JJ, Kao SC, Vallely MP, van Zandwijk N, Reid G. The impact of hemolysis on cell-free microRNA Biomarkers. Frontiers in Genetics. 2013;4:94.

[179] Blondal T, Jensby Nielsen S, Baker A, Andreasen D, Mouritzen P, Wrang Teilum M, et al. Assessing sample and miRNA profile quality in serum and plasma or other biofluids. Methods (San Diego, Calif). 2013;59(1):S1–6.

[180] Costa MC, Leitão LA, Enguita JF. MicroRNA profiling in plasma or serum using quantitative RT-PCR. In: Alvarez L, Nourbakhsh M, editors. RNA Mapping: Methods and Protocols, Methods in Molecular Biology. 1182. New York: Springer Science and Business Media; 2014. p. 121–9.

[181] Teruel R, Perez-Sanchez C, Corral J, Herranz MT, Perez-Andreu V, Saiz E, et al. Identification of miRNAs as potential modulators of tissue factor expression in patients with systemic lupus erythematosus and antiphospholipid syndrome. Journal of Thrombosis and Haemostasis. 2011;9(10):1985–92.